CALVARY HOSPITAL

MODEL FOR PALLIATIVE CARE IN ADVANCED CANCER

James E. Cimino, M.D., Michael J. Brescia, M.D., Editors

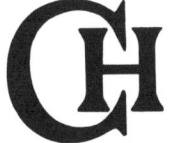

This book has been underwritten through the unrestricted Langer Foundation Grant given to Calvary Hospital's Palliative Care Institute.

Copyright © 1998 by

CALVARY HOSPITAL

Library of Congress Catalog Card Number:
98-67495
ISBN 0-930194-98-5

PUBLISHED BY:
The Palliative Care Institute
Calvary Hospital
1740 Eastchester Rd.
Bronx, N.Y.

Drug therapy is an important part of palliative care. A list of commonly used medications with the usual dosage schedule appears throughout the text. However, no liability is assumed for typographic or other errors and before any of these drugs are prescribed it is recommended that current prescribing information be reviewed in package inserts. The opinions expressed in this book are those of each of the authors and not necessarily those of Calvary Hospital.

Printed at I.P.O Graphics, Inc.
Merrick, N.Y.

CALVARY HOSPITAL - MODEL FOR PALLIATIVE CARE IN ADVANCED CANCER

CONTENTS

FOREWORD x
    Frank Calamari

INTRODUCTION 1
    James E. Cimino, Michael J. Brescia

I. RELIEF OF SYMPTOMS

   1. Pain 3
       Michael J. Brescia

   2. Non-Cancer Related Pain in End of Life Cancer Patient 7
       James E. Cimino

   3. The Use of Intraspinal Infusion Pumps 10
       Carol Kyriannis

   4. Pain Management in the Substance Abuser 13
       Lyla J. Correoso

   5. Fatigue 17
       Charles Kyriannis

   6. Dyspnea I 21
       Michael J. Brescia

   7. Dyspnea II - Special Considerations: Malignant Pleural Effusions;
     Pulse Oximetry 25
       Joseph Casinio

   8. Gastrointestinal Malignant Obstruction 29
       Michael J. Brescia

   9. Nausea and Vomiting 33
       Rekha Mehta

  10. Seizures 38
       Antonios Vlantis

  11. Delirium and Depression 42
       Robert A. Brescia

II. SPECIAL CONSIDERATIONS IN THE PALLIATIVE CARE SETTING

1. Intercurrent Diseases 45
   James E. Cimino

2. Chemotherapy: Its Place in Palliative Care:
   Breast, Prostate, Pancreas, Multiple Myeloma 48
   David I. Wollner

   Lung, Colorectal, Non-Hodgkins Lymphomas 51
   Devmani Jaitly

3. Radiotherapy 56
   Flora Mincer

4. Hypercalcemia 58
   Michael Eufemio

5. AIDS 63
   Dial Hewlett, Jr.

6. Urological Care 68
   Richard Bard

7. Cardiovascular Problems 72
   Sharad Jaitley

8. CPR and DNR 77
   Gail Chrzanowski

9. Blood Transfusion Practices 80
   Cynthia Collins and Michael J. Brescia

10. Physical Therapy 83
    Edward Casey

11. Diagnostic Radiology 86
    Arnold Berrett

III. NURSING

1. Theory and Philosophy and the Cancer Care
   Technician Program 89
   Patricia Tennell

v

      2. Enterostomal Therapy Services 95
          Catherine Kalinski and Mary Schnepf

IV. **NUTRITION**

      1. Cachexia of Cancer 98
          James E. Cimino

      2. Calvary Hospital's Nurturing Tradition 102
          Elizabeth D. Looney

      3. Nutrition Support and Non-Abandonment 108
          James E. Cimino

V. **PHARMACY**

      1. Pharmaceutical Services and
         Concentrated Morphine 114
          John Grom

      2. Commonly Used Medications 117
          Barbara Romeo

      3. Drug and Food Interactions 129
          Rick Tota

VI. **SOCIAL WORK** 135
          Barbara Guilfoyle and Debbie Feldman

VII. **THERAPEUTIC RECREATION AND LIFE AFFIRMATION** 140
          Nanette Vallecillo

VIII. **VOLUNTEERS** 144
          Mary Ann Gulla

IX. **PATIENT/FAMILY ADVOCACY** 146
          Joan Caldano

X. **PASTORAL CARE** 151
          Mary Teresa O'Neill

XI. **BEREAVEMENT SUPPORT SERVICES** 154
          Catherine R. Seeley

XII.	HOME CARE	158
	Carol Townsend and Anthony R. Riario	
XIII.	THOUGHTS ON:	

1. Euthanasia 161
   James E. Cimino

2. Assisted Suicide 167
   Michael J. Brescia

3. Perceptions: Depersonalizations, Reflections --
   Literary Correlates in Palliative Medicine 170
   Anthony R. Riario

4. Expenditures for Dying Patients: Too Much or Not Enough? 175
   Frank A. Calamari

CONTRIBUTORS: CALVARY HOSPITAL STAFF

Richard Bard, M.D., F.A.C.S.
Attending Medical Staff
Associate Clinical Professor, Urology
Cornell University Medical College

Arnold Berrett, M.D.
Director, Radiology
Associate Clinical Professor of Radiology
New York Medical College

Michael J. Brescia, M.D.
Medical Director
Clinical Assistant Professor of Medicine
New York Medical College

Robert A. Brescia, M.D.
Director, Psychiatric Services

Frank A. Calamari, M.B.A.
President, Chief Executive Officer

S. Joan Caldano, F.S.P., M.S.Ed.
Patient/Family Advocate

Edward Casey, M.D.
Director, Physical Therapy

Joseph Casino, M.D.
Attending Medical Staff
Attending Pulmonary & Critical Care
Sound Shore Medical Center
Assistant Clinical Professor, Medicine
New York Medical College

Gail Chrzanowski, M.D.
Attending Medical Staff

James E. Cimino, M.D., F.A.C.P.
Director, Palliative Care Institute
Clinical Professor of Medicine
New York Medical College

Lyla J. Correoso, M.D.
Attending Medical Staff

Michael Eufemio, M.D.
Attending Medical Staff
Chief of Endocrinology, Soundshore Medical Center. Clinical Assistant Professor of Medicine, New York Medical College

Deborah Feldman, M.S.W., A.C.S.W.
Director, Department of Family Care

John Grom, R.Ph., M.S., M.B.A.
Assistant Administrator, Clinical Support Services, Director of Pharmaceutical Services, Affiliate Assistant Clinical Professor, St. John's University

Barbara Guilfoyle, M.S.W., A.C.S.W.
Assistant Administrator for Patient and Family Support Services.
Director, Social Work Services

Mary Ann Gulla, B.A.
Director, Volunteers

Dial Hewlett, Jr., M.D., F.A.C.P.
Consultant, Infectious Disease
Associate Medical Director of Clinical & Scientific Affairs, Pfizer Corporation
Associate Professor of Clinical Medicine
New York Medical College

Devmani Jaitly, M.D.
Attending Medical Staff

Sharad C. Jaitly, M.D., F.A.C.C.
Attending Medical Staff
Cardiologist
Cardiothoracic & Vascular Group
New Haven, CT

Catherine Kalinski, R.N., A.A.S., C.E.T.N.
Enterostomal Therapist

Carol Kyriannis, M.D.
Attending Medical Staff

Charles Kyriannis, M.D.
Attending Medical Staff

Elizabeth D. Looney, C.S.J., M.A., R.D., C.D.N.
Director, Nutritional Services

Rekha Mehta, M.D.
Attending Medical Staff
Attending Gastroenterologist
Sound Shore Medical Center

Flora Mincer, M.D.
Radiation Oncologist
Associate Professor of Radiation
  Oncology, Emeritus
Albert Einstein College of Medicine

Mary T. O'Neill, M.A.
Assistant Administrator/Director
Pastoral Services

Anthony R. Riario, M.D.
Attending Medical Staff
Consultant to Home Health Agency
Clinical Assistant Professor of Medicine,
New York Medical College

Barbara Romeo, Pharm.D.
Supervisor, Clinical Pharmaceutical
Services

Mary Schnepf, R.N., R.N.C., M.P.,H.E.T.
Enterostomal Therapist

Catherine Seeley, M.A.
Director, Bereavement Services

Patricia Tennell, R.N., M.P.H., C.N.A.A.
Associate Administrator/Director of Nursing

Rick Tota, R.Ph., M.S.
Associate Director, Pharmaceutical
Services. Preceptor, St. John's University

Carol Townsend, R.N., B.S.N., M.P.S.
Administrator, Certified Home
Health Agency

Nanette Vallecillo, C.T.R.S., M.S.
Director, Therapeutic Recreation

Antonios Vlantis, M.D.
Attending Medical Staff

David I. Wollner, M.D.
Attending Medical Staff
Assistant Professor of Medicine
Albert Einstein College of Medicine

DEDICATION

We want to dedicate this book to the founders, the trustees, our patients, their families and their caregivers, our staff, past and present without whom none of this could have happened.

Acknowledgments

We want to thank Ms. Peggy Looney, Assistant Administrator for Professional Services, for her encouragement and help, not only for this book, but for her twenty-four years of friendship.

Sr. Elizabeth Looney, Director of Nutritional Services, not only nourished our bodies and souls for twenty-three years, but was particularly helpful and generous in her review of some of the manuscripts in this book.

Ms. Sheri Sussman, our Managing Editor, was a pleasure to work with as she guided us through this project and we thank her.

Ms. Maryann Santarsiero, Assistant to the Director of the Palliative Care Institute, worked relentlessly typing and correcting the entire manuscript. How she survived and tolerated working with us and the other authors is a wonderment. Maryann, our heartfelt thanks.

FOREWORD
Frank Calamari

The great transformation of American health care into a proprietary, managed care driven system is a process of which we are all aware and one that is well documented in most forms of academic and professional literature. However, another powerful process is also occurring within these economic and social changes that will serve to either re-anchor our moral and ethical moorings or hasten the process of our losing hold of them. This movement involves society's dealing with the concepts of physician-assisted suicide and euthanasia, coupled with health care's long overdue recognition of the need for palliative care directed toward terminal patients and members of their family. This area of care has been ignored and considered an "academic backwater" that made respected clinicians uncomfortable in its midst and condescending toward its challenges and impact. It is no surprise, therefore, that our society rushes to "Kevorkian" solutions for our desperately sick loved ones when American clinical care has so little to offer.

Within this general vacuum of adequacy there, lies great hope and direction for the future. Throughout the pages of this book you will come to understand Calvary Hospital and its Program of Care; an example of caring and compassion that has evolved over the past one hundred years, and is now ready to provide the guidance to the American health care system for the delivery of palliative care to patients and their families.

As with many clinical endeavors, top notch qualitative and quantitative medical and nursing care is a sine qua non. Those patients whose bodies have betrayed them and whose spirits and emotions are being racked to the very core cannot be short changed. Because these patients cannot be cured, we must guard against a "capital acquisition" mentality whereby we are reluctant to properly treat them because their broken bodies may not be able to be "fixed." Hospice programs in our country certainly have a role to play in the care of some of these patients, however, automatically referring people into home hospice programs with an ill prepared family support system, must not be forced upon us as a "one-size-fits-all" (cheap) solution for the delivery of palliative care.

If these clinical changes were evolving independent of the other changes in health care, their adoption alone would be a daunting and grueling process. However, in the context of a health care system changing into one being driven more and more by profits than by caring, it makes the task extremely difficult.

This book will provide a guide for academicians and clinicians committed to making palliative care part of the American health care system. Its words are also a testimony and a tribute to the original founders, the past contributors, and the current staff of Calvary Hospital.

INTRODUCTION
James E. Cimino and Michael J. Brescia

This book represents Calvary Hospital's clinical program across the entire spectrum of patient care. Each discipline involved in the patient's care has some unique contribution to make. It is divided into sections that consist of individual essays. Although these essays express the individual authors' opinions and observations, they also reflect the Calvary program as a whole.

The book begins by addressing symptoms because symptom relief is the foundation of palliative care. The topics that follow, discuss those disciplines which further embrace this model of care. Although ethics is not addressed as a separate subject, it is embodied in a number of essays, particularly those dealing with pain, dyspnea, nutrition, special medical problems, euthanasia, assisted suicide, and administrative considerations.

Calvary Hospital is a modern two-hundred bed facility caring for advanced cancer patients. Located in the northeast section of the Bronx in New York City, it is operated by the New York Roman Catholic Archdiocese. Calvary earned a reputation for compassionate and skillful control of patients' symptoms long before palliative and hospice care became popular disciplines. The foundations for this care are kindness and clinical competence. Both qualities are evident in the philosophy of "non-abandonment" of the patient and the cooperation among all of the caregivers.

In 1899, eleven Catholic widows were organized as the Women of Calvary by Annie Blount Storrs. Her inspiration was a similar group, the *Dames de Calvaire* from Lyon, France, founded by Madame Jeanne Garnier in 1842. Along with other women, Madame Garnier opened their first hospital. Subsequently, their work spread to Paris, Marseilles, Saint Etienne, Rouen, Bordeaux, Brussels, and Jerusalem. It was in Brussels that Mrs. Storrs became acquainted with the Dames de Calvaire. The New York women cared for indigent and terminal patients in two private houses on Perry Street in Manhattan until 1915 when they moved to the Bronx. The Women of Calvary were assisted by the Dominican Sisters of Blauvelt until 1958. That same year, Catherine McParlan, the last of the founders died. The work was continued by the Dominican Sisters of the Sick Poor until 1974. Since then, a lay administration has led the program.

In the early 1960s, the medical program was formalized. In 1962, the Cancer Care Technician (CCT) Program was developed. The CCTs are para-professionals who deliver hands-on nursing care under the direction of the professional nursing staff. Calvary was recognized and accredited as a hospital by the Joint Commission on Accreditation of Healthcare Organizations (JCAHO) in 1965. In the fall of 1997, it **received its third consecutive three-year accreditation with *commendation*** from the JCAHO.

Protocols and procedures used at Calvary Hospital are much the same as one expects to find in any excellent hospital. What is different is the consistent and dedicated commitment to this special mission when these procedures of caring for the advanced cancer patients are put into practice.

Our goal is to help the patient live comfortably and usefully until life ends. It is important to think of the patient as *living,* rather than *dying.* Our care is patient rather than disease oriented. We are dedicated to the relief of all discomforts and to the belief that symptom control is not an excuse for careless medical management. We treat the patient near death as a living human being. The care is not a monopoly of any one discipline. Everyone involved in the patient's care makes some unique contribution. The family is part of the unit of care and is given exceptional attention throughout the patient's illness.

When someone is hospitalized, it is a frightening experience. Non-abandonment means removing this fear. It also means communicating, being available, showing genuine concern, ensuring continuity of care, and keeping promises. This is the theme that connects us to our patients, their families, and to each other. Hopefully, this is reflected in this book.

PAIN
Michael J. Brescia

Pain is a complex combination of factors affecting the patient and presents in various ways. Patients can suffer from diverse effects of pain including spiritual, mental, emotional, physical, and familial pain.

Physical Abuse

Physical pain can be due to the disease itself as well as the physical abuse of a protracted disease such as prolonged bed rest, malnutrition and general diminution in nursing and medical care associated with long term terminal disease.

Physical abuse includes the failure to provide personal hygiene and encompasses care of hair, nails, mouth, and dentures.

Patients may present with multiple or single decubiti which in themselves can produce significant symptoms.

There is also failure of internal hygiene including fecal impaction which occurs in approximately 10% of patients arriving at Calvary Hospital. Improper bowel hygiene is frequently associated with nausea, vomiting, and loss of appetite. This is not generally recognized and treated.

Additional failures of internal hygiene include urinary retention and oral and vaginal fungal infections. Patients with colostomies, ileostomies and nephrostomies frequently have failure of stoma function. This results in drainage of liquids that are rich in enzymes or irritants causing digestion and breakdown of surrounding skin at the exit of tubes.

Fistulae of rectal, vaginal and cutaneous origin require an enormous effort to control both odor and skin damage. Frequently, the development of a fistula can signal a better prognosis since there is venting of obstructed bowel or another viscous organ which may allow the patient to be more comfortable. Profuse drainage and the resulting skin breakdown, incontinence and difficult odor control can make this a disastrous complication.

The control of physical abuse requires intense nursing care and includes enterostomal specialists and Cancer Care Technicians in addition to the staff nurse.

Physical Pain Therapy

Physical pain therapy can be divided into non-opioid and opioid therapy and further divided by classes of drugs. Among the non-opioid drugs are the non-steroidal anti-inflammatory drugs (NSAIDs) which are used predominantly for the control of bone pain. (NSAIDs have a very rapid ceiling dose.) Effective use of NSAIDs at Calvary Hospital has not been high. These patients should have, along with the use of NSAIDs, the inclusion of misoprostol. This prostaglandin II analog assists with the formation of mucous and the prevention of massive bleeding which can be a significant complication, especially in older patients, patients with gastrointestinal malignancies, and those with a history of peptic ulcer disease.

Opioids

Opioids are the most frequently used analgesics at Calvary Hospital. These are codeine, oxycodone with or without acetaminophen, hydromorphone, levorphanol, methadone, morphine, and fentanyl (Duragesic Patch). Oxycodone and morphine make up the vast bulk of opiate usage.

Routes of Administration

Routes of administration are oral, intranasal, sublingual, buccal, transdermal, rectal and parenteral. Parenteral include subcutaneous, intramuscular, intravenous, intravenous bolus, intravenous continuous infusion, intermittent or continuous subcutaneous infusions, epidural, and intrathecal. Major routes of administration of narcotics at Calvary Hospital are oral, subcutaneous, and intravenous. Intravenous can be by the use of a patient controlled analgesia (PCA) pump or a regular intravenous continuous pump. IV bolus is generally not used except in severe cases of uncontrolled pain and severe instances of dyspnea. At Calvary Hospital, the epidural route appears to be successful over shorter periods of time. Side effects of opioid administration are usually temporary and preventable when the physician attentively monitors the patient. Opioids offer the best modality for control of symptoms in terminal disease.

Common Side Effects

Constipation is prevented with general bowel hygiene and routine use of laxatives. Nausea and vomiting are usually minor problems because they are transient and can be controlled with routine antiemetic therapy. Urinary retention can occur but, if present, may be related to other complicating diseases.

When respiratory depression occurs it is rarely prolonged. Sedation, which may or may not be desirable, varies greatly and can usually be resolved to the patient's satisfaction. If sedation is persistent, it may be related to other sedating medications given simultaneously. Confusion and delirium may occur during opioid therapy and are greater when drugs with long half lives such as levorphanol and methadone are used. Confusion and delirium can be treated with anti-psychotic therapy.

Meperidine is a poor drug for pain control. It has highly toxic metabolites and a rapid development of tolerance. It is only used at Calvary Hospital when there is a true allergy to other opioids or when a patient insists on its use.

Narcotic Dosing Protocol

Morphine allergies are rare and one must be extremely cautious before such an effective drug is denied a patient on the basis of allergy.

In general, patients on narcotic therapy who can swallow, are treated with oxycodone, 5-10 mg every 4 hours and every 2 hours as necessary. If there is only a partial effect, we generally proceed to another oral opioid such as hydromorphone or morphine immediate release. Hydromorphone and oral morphine can be given on a similar schedule. A routine dose every 4 - 6 hours and every 2 hours prn. If there is only partial analgesia, oral dosage is increased. (Refer to tables in pharmacy section.)

Morphine sulfate therapy can be given subcutaneously and is the parenteral drug of choice. Calvary Hospital compounds morphine at 50mg per ml. This permits the administration of very small volumes. Size 29g needles are used with minimal discomfort. Morphine 5 mg to 50 mg can be given routinely every 4 to 6 hours and more importantly, as rescue at the patient's request. If the patient requires very frequent dosing or has an objection to needles, a morphine sulfate continuous infusion can be used. Rescue IV or SQ morphine is also available. If morphine sulfate concentrate is not available, a patient would be a candidate for continuous IV infusion much sooner. The amount of morphine infusion is related to the response obtained and not to any maximum dose allowed. In general, 500 mg of morphine by continuous IV infusion will be an effective analgesia in almost all cases, but the need for 4000 mg is not rare.

Neuropathic Pain

Neuropathic pain is often treated with tricyclic compounds particularly amitriptyline in addition to the standard analgesics. This treatment protocol has not generally proven successful with Calvary Hospital patients. The number of complications due to this drug can be explained by the debilitated state of our patients. Anticholinergic effects -- arrhythmias, urinary retention -- frequently produce more problems than benefit. Anticonvulsants and steroids are also useful for neuropathic pain. Whenever pain is perceived to be due to an inflammatory mechanism, steroids may be used in high doses for short periods of time. If a positive effect is obtained, the steroid is lowered to the lowest effective maintenance dose. Examples include large bulky node compressions which may regress with therapy or reduction of edema and swelling in confined areas, e.g., spinal canal.

Summary

The greatest cause of failure of pain control has been the unwillingness to use appropriate doses of opioids. When opioids are used, the physician must continuously monitor and evaluate their effectiveness and individualize both dose and schedule. The patient's symptoms must be acknowledged and treated. Addiction is rare and patients and families should be reassured when this issue is raised. The addition of concentrated morphine has made the subcutaneous route a very valuable route freeing the patient from IV lines and allowing a more extended life style while in the final months of life. Other considerations of pain control and specific dosage schedules are covered in subsequent chapters.

Failure to recognize and treat other modalities of suffering will not offer successful palliation in advanced cancer.

Reference

1. World Health Organization (WHO) Analgesic Ladder 1990; Clinical Practice Guidelines, No. 9, p 41-45.

NON-CANCER RELATED PAIN IN END-OF-LIFE CANCER PATIENTS
James E. Cimino

The emphasis on management of pain in the cancer patient during the past 20 years has not only called attention to the lack of skillful pain management in these patients, but in all suffering individuals. This discussion demonstrates that the etiology of pain can be separate from a patient's cancer. The etiologies of pain are as numerous as humankind's many diseases. In spite of the existential nature of pain and the difficulty in defining it, cancer patients can be as frustrated as physicians in describing it. My understanding is that pain is a subjective, unpleasant feeling due to changes or tissue damage.

The word "terminal" is usually applied to end-of-life cancer patients. Because of the growth of hospice and its use of the category, a terminal prognosis generally refers to approximately 6 months of remaining life. Unfortunately, the difficulty with this definition is that we are no more likely to accurately predict a 6-month prognosis in patients as we are in adequately understanding the severity of a patient's pain.

We must depend upon the patient to tell us how unpleasant the pain is and how we should weigh the importance of limited life expectancy against the patient's acceptance of a recommended treatment. For example, we may decide that a patient's prognosis is more likely measured in days or weeks rather than months, but only he or she can guide us as to the importance these time frames bear in determining a treatment benefit in relation to the burden the patient is willing to accept.

It is likely that if we can establish the cause of a non-cancer pain, we will have greater success in relieving it. This may prove to be one of the greatest challenges we face in end-of-life cancer patients. Too often caregivers attribute all the discomfort to the underlying malignancy. That can be the beginning of the "abandonment syndrome" which interferes with our objective and diagnostic acumen.

The basic principles of pain management are no different, whatever the etiology. First, establish a cause, then assess the pain using the various scales available or by the patient's subjective evaluation, describing it as "moderate," "severe," "not too bad," or "the worst I ever had," etc. Then choose the appropriate therapy based on cause and the pain's general characteristics. For instance, pain may be somatic and related to musculoskeletal abnormalities and inflammatory tissue damage. It may be visceral due to pressure and/or distention of internal organs or it may be neuropathic, due to damage of a nerve itself rather than damage to tissue innervated by the nerve. These principles are the same as those we apply in the advanced cancer patient. If we can treat the underlying disease, then we should do so.

Generally the difference between cancer pain and non-cancer related pain is that we can't do much for the underlying cancer. As a result, pain relief becomes paramount and adverse side effects, though addressed, are less important, including the possibility of shortening life. There is also less anxiety about opioid addiction in those with a limited life expectancy. It is preferable to use a non-opioid analgesic with or without adjuvant therapy, but if it produces no benefit, then the addition of a weak opioid, with or without an adjuvant, followed by a stronger opioid can be used. In opioid use, constipation and nausea must be anticipated and preferably addressed even before these side effects occur.

The principles of analgesic therapy are generally agreed upon.[1] Oral administration should be used whenever possible. Medication should be given around the clock in anticipation of pain breakthrough. The non-opioid analgesics generally are acetaminophen, aspirin, and non-steroidal anti-inflammatory drugs. Weak opioids are those with an analgesic ceiling, meaning that at a certain dosage, they will not increase analgesia but can cause an increase in toxicity. An example of a weak opioid is codeine. The strong opioids are: morphine, fentanyl, hydromorphone, levorphanol, methadone, and oxycodone (probably very close in analgesic effectiveness to morphine). The so-called "strong" opioids can be used at whatever dose it takes to relieve pain. The side effects and toxicity of these drugs do not necessarily escalate as the dose is increased.

Neuropathic pain is preferably treated with tricyclic antidepressant medications, anticonvulsants, and sometimes anxiolytics. Other adjuvants that may be useful are muscle relaxants such as cyclobenzaprine (Flexeril) and at times corticosteroids. An anesthetic agent such as mexiletine has also been recommended but I have no experience with it. Psycho-stimulants such as ritalin (methylphenidate) and pemoline (cylert) can reduce opioid-induced sedation (and may even alleviate depression).

This is a description of one patient who typified the problem of what occurs when we succumb to the mindset initiated by an end-of-life diagnosis of cancer. This patient lived with significant discomfort for much longer than was reasonable. He was an 80-year-old man with adenocarcinoma of the lung. He had undergone an extensive work-up and later, exploratory surgery. The lesion was deemed inoperable and he received radiotherapy. This patient's course was complicated by atrial fibrillation with rapid ventricular response and congestive heart failure. Digoxin and anticoagulants were started. Some weeks after the patient was discharged from the hospital, he developed herpes zoster (shingles) infection overlying the lower lumbar area. Herpes zoster results from reactivation of varicella viruses that remain dormant for the life of an individual. Although it may begin with nerve pain, it is shortly followed with blister-like lesions in the skin areas innervated by the affected nerve group. It appears to be more common in elderly and immuno-compromised patients. Anywhere from 10-20% of patients develop a persistent severe pain that usually lasts for 1 to 2 months but in some cases, persists for many months to years. It can be treated with a high dose of acyclovir, and a recent study shows that adding amitriptyline may decrease the incidence and/or severity of the post herpetic neuralgia.[2] It is not uncommon for patients with advanced lung cancer and a shortened life expectancy not to be given the benefit of this aggressive care. This patient's neuralgia subsided considerably after a month. One month later, he experienced back pain in the same general vicinity and it was thought to be due to a worsening of the herpetic neuralgia. This resulted in delay of diagnostic studies. Subsequently, x-rays revealed suspicion of metastatic lesions in the lumbar vertebrae and pelvic rim on the same side as the pain. The patient was treated initially with mild analgesics, without anti-inflammatory agents because of the fear of bleeding while on coumadin maintenance therapy. The pain was then treated with the addition of opioids. A further work-up, including CT-scan, revealed a herniated intervertebral disc. The patient was managed with increasing doses of opioids and manifested periods of significant confusion, mild nausea, and severe constipation. These symptoms resulted in the addition of other medications that further complicated the case. It was then decided to discontinue the coumadin therapy and place the patient on a non-steroidal anti-inflammatory agent, which resulted in considerable improvement. Although opioids could not be withdrawn completely, the patient was able to participate in physical therapy and ambulate for the first time in over a month. Amelioration of the pain also resulted in the decrease of other medications needed to treat side effects. All of this occurred during a period of 3 months, and more than 2 years after the patient had been thought to have a life prognosis of less than 6 months and categorized as terminal.

There are numerous examples of how one can delay and therefore affect discomfort levels of patients who are diagnosed as terminally ill. Some examples are: patients with bone metastases who develop arthritis, those with intraabdominal metastases who suffer from cholelithiasis or renal colic, patients with intraabdominal carcinoma with bowel obstruction secondary to a more mundane fecal impaction, or the dilemma of how aggressive to be in treating long bone fractures. Only the patient understands the severity of the discomfort and the meaning of the remaining days or weeks of life.

Another challenging problem is the evaluation and management of pain in cognitively-impaired individuals We need to learn to interpret the moaning, the groaning, the grimaces, and the restlessness of these patients. Often our cancer care technicians and nurses are able to understand the meaning of these gestures. Or they may be understood only by close relatives. The caregivers must pay attention and listen. It is never wrong to treat these patients with analgesics as a therapeutic trial.

Ultimately we must return to the evaluation of benefits and burdens. How much of a burden is the patient willing to endure in order to obtain pain relief or other symptoms of suffering. This is the same standard we apply in all our practice when it is done well. When a patient perceives a treatment as beneficial and that it causes little or no burden, it is a rare patient who would refuse and the rare caregiver that would withhold it. However, as the likelihood of benefit decreases and the burden increases, it is then that concern for the patient and our wisdom are tested. This is when diagnostic acumen and experience reveal the value of the concerned and competent caregiver.

References

1. World Health Organization (WHO), 1990. The analgesic ladder clinical practice guideline. No. 9, Management of Cancer Pain. U.S. Dept. of Health & Human Services Pub. No. 94-0592.

2. Bowsher D. The effects of pre-emptive treatment of postherapeutic neuralgia with amitriptyline: a randomized, double-blind, placebo-controlled trial. J Pain Symp Manag 1997; 13: pp 327-331.

THE USE OF INTRASPINAL INFUSION PUMPS
Carol Kyriannis

Intraspinal opioids by an implanted drug administration device has grown in popularity and has become an accepted form of therapy for intractable cancer and non-cancer pain.[1,2,3] For the most part, the existing studies are uncontrolled and retrospective with only small numbers of patients. Clinicians, therefore, are forced to base decisions about intrathecal morphine or another narcotic or mixtures of narcotic-anesthetic agents, on evidence from case reports and limited series of patients. Questions remain regarding the most effective method of screening that may predict long term response, choice of narcotic and anesthetic agent for a specific type of pain, development of tolerance, dose change over time, and prevalence of adverse effects.

The development of continuous infusion pumps for pain control was made possible by technological advances since 1985. The most common devises consist of continuous administration of medication with a mechanism by which the patient can administer bolus doses for break-through pain. In the early 1900s, local anesthetics, e.g., cocaine were administered in the epidural space for analgesia. In 1949, drugs were placed in the spinal canal for post-op analgesia. In the 1970s, widespread clinical use of anesthetics and morphine occurred only after opioid receptors in the spinal cord were identified.

During 1997, thirty-one patients were managed with epidural and four patients with intrathecal infusions. These were discontinued only if complications occurred.

Physiology

The epidural space is located between the outer surface of the dura mater and the bony walls of the spinal canal. It contains nerve roots, fat, spinal avenues, lymphatic channels, and a valveless venous system which can influence the action of narcotics. Epidural fat contains a rich network of capillaries and provides a large surface area for drug uptake. Direct access to the brain is possible for agents injected epidurally. Potential CNS toxicity is possible if a drug is administered at a high dose. This is due to the existence of the continuous valveless vascular connection.

Mechanism and Sites of Action

Opioids selectively block pain conduction that occupy specific pain receptors in the spinal cord. Local anesthetics provide analgesia by axonal membrane blockade and also produce non-selective sympathetic (sensory and motor) blockade in addition to analgesia.

An opioid-local anesthetic mixture should provide an additive analgesic effect. Lipid solubility of a narcotic (drug) is the most important determinant in effecting the drugs onset of action, duration of action and its dermatomal spread. Morphine and hydromorphone (lower lipid solubility) have a slower onset of action, a longer duration of action and a greater dermatomal spread than fentanyl and methadone (higher lipid solubility). Morphine is used epidurally, but gives more effective pain control if given intrathecally, especially if intractable pain exists along much of the spine. This is due to morphine being less lipid soluble and takes advantage of the concept of "Rostral Flow" or "Rostral Spread." Once morphine is in the subarachnoid space the drug is carried away from the site of injection. Fentanyl is 10 times more effective than morphine when administered in this manner.

The appropriate conversion of spinal morphine dose to parenteral morphine dose is as follows:

Epidural morphine dose = 24 hour morphine parenteral dose divided by 10

Intrathecal morphine dose = epidural dose divided by 10.

Local anesthetics such as Bupivacaine and Lidocaine are also used to enhance and act via other receptors to control pain. Lipid solubility is the primary determinant of the potency of local anesthetics. Lidocaine has an intermediate anesthetic potency and lipophilicity. Bupivacaine has high anesthetic potency and lipophilicity.

Complications

The complications of spinal medication administration are: headache, infection of epidural space, bleeding of epidural space, and catheter migration after placement.

In recent articles which reviewed a series of intrathecal administration, one in five had catheter-related problems, e.g., kinking.

Adverse drug reactions to opioids administered intraspinally are: respiratory depression, pruritus (cause unknown), urinary retention, nausea/vomiting, cardiovascular, and excessive sedation. Additional adverse reactions of intraspinally administered local anesthetics are: urinary retention, hypotension, numbness, and motor weakness. During 1997, five patients were admitted with epidural catheters in place and four patients with intrathecal catheters. These catheters and pumps are maintained as long as they are functioning properly.

Conclusion

When considering the indications for use of intraspinal infusion pumps, one must take into account the type of tumor, the stage of disease, the mental status of the patient, the presence of intractable pain -- location, radiation, and type of pain, and the performance status of the patient. Consultation with an anesthesiologist is essential.

References

1. Waldman SD. The role of spinal opioids in the management of cancer pain. J Pain Symptom Manag 1990;5(3):163-168.

2. Muir MR, Sullivan FL, Dear G, et al. Monitoring practices following epidural analgesics for pain management: A follow-up survey. J Pain Symptom Manage 1997;14(1):pp 36-44.

3. Krames ES. Intrathecal infusional therapies for intractable pain: patient management guidelines. J Pain Symptom Manage 1993;8(1): pp 36-46.

PAIN MANAGEMENT IN THE SUBSTANCE ABUSER
Lyla J. Correoso

Substance abusers are one group of patients that are at risk of being under treated for pain. These patients may suffer needlessly due to poorly informed caregivers. The patients themselves are an obstacle to receiving adequate pain relief. There are also legal barriers that impair adequate treatment of pain in general. Here is an exploration of some of these barriers.

Barriers

Despite many advances in medicine, some old myths still persist about narcotic usage. Many health care professionals still believe that patients can easily become addicted to opioids. A study of 12,000 cancer patients revealed that only three became addicted and these patients were considered to have a prior problem with chemical dependency.[1] In patients with an addiction history, there is a great fear that the patient is looking for drugs and is indeed manipulating the health care professional. With this in mind, many practitioners are excessively scrutinizing before using appropriate narcotics for these patients. The reality is that an experienced, unintimidated, and compassionate professional is what the patient needs.

In 1961, one hundred World governments devised the Single Convention on Narcotic Drugs which serves as the framework for all narcotic legislation from national to the state level. The preamble of the Convention is "the ratifying governments recognize that the medical use of narcotic drugs continues to be indispensable for the relief of pain and suffering and that adequate provision must be made to ensure the availability of narcotic drugs for such purposes." The second part deals with drug addiction, but the Convention put the concerns of health over the concerns related to addiction and abuse. After that Convention, the Controlled Substance Act was started as the US Federal Narcotic Control Law. In theory, it states that the "concerns of law enforcement agencies have to be balanced with concerns from the health community." In some states the use of triplicate prescriptions was started to control the use of narcotics. However, it was shown through an American Medical Association study that the states that utilized triplicate forms had a higher rate of drug abuse than those that did not.[2] In addition, the use of narcotics for cancer patients decreased and less potent analgesics were being used. The use of triplicates meant to improve the surveillance by drug enforcement agencies of health care professionals and pharmacists, did not lend itself to good pain management. In addition, many local pharmacies are reluctant to carry narcotics because of fear of robbery.

Another major barrier to good pain control is the professionals' and the public's perceptions of narcotics. Far too few professionals understand the difference between physical tolerance and true addiction.

Opioids

For substance abusers with cancer or AIDS, pain should be assessed as in any other patient and then the World Health Organization (WHO) analgesic ladder[3] should be followed. Depending on the severity of the pain - weak, moderate, or strong opioids are indicated. Codeine, oxycodone, hydromorphone, morphine, levodromoran, fentanyl, and even methadone may be used. There is no contraindication to using an intravenous drip (IV) or Patient Controlled Analgesic (PCA) pump, if it is appropriate. Adjuvant drugs may be used. The mixed agonist-antagonist class of drugs should not be used. This group includes pentazocine, butorphanol, buprenorphine, dezocine and nalbuphine. The problems that may arise include the possible precipitation of severe withdrawal. There is also a ceiling effect of the partial agonist, thus the patient may not get adequate analgesia. Another drug to be avoided is meperidine. The active metabolite, normeperidine can accumulate when high doses are used, particularly when in the presence of renal impairment. Normeperidine is a CNS stimulant and its accumulation may result in tremors, jerking, twitching, and ultimately grand mal seizures.

Dosing

It is important to relieve the pain. This requires increasing the dose of opioid until the patient reports satisfactory pain relief or until unmanageable side effects occur. Patients with a history of chemical dependance may require significantly higher doses of narcotics. They may have built up a tolerance when they were either on illicit drugs or on a methadone maintenance program. This will not only apply to opioids, but to any sedatives that may be needed in conjunction with the narcotic. Should you suspect that a patient has developed an overdose, the use of naloxone should be used cautiously. These patients have experienced withdrawal in the past and are terrified of going through it again.

Management Guidelines

Patients who are substance abusers are separated into three groups - active users, Methadone Maintenance Treatment Program (MMTP) participants, and rehabilitated or recovered abusers. Each group has its own individual problems and requirements. An active abuser may be using illegal drugs to achieve pain control because no one will listen or believe the severity of the pain. The MMTP patient may want to be maintained on the methadone program dose in addition to the pain relieving dose because of the fear of withdrawal. The recovered abuser is usually more reluctant to use narcotics because of the fear of becoming addicted again. For these patients, it becomes most difficult. They may experience "nodding out," slurred speech, or become clock watchers. To these patients and their families this may seem as though they are once again addicted. In reality these behaviors are not unusual for any patient using narcotics. Once the patient has used the medication for a few days these events dissipate. If the patient is a clock watcher, whether substance abuser or not, this may be an indication that the pain is not adequately controlled.

The staff's interpretation of the patient's pain complaints are crucial to successful management in this patient population. Lack of trust in the patient's pain report can lead to the undoing of patient/health care professional relationship as well as fuel the fears of the family. When beginning the care of a patient, it is useful to review the philosophy of care with the family. The mission of the institution and the goals of care should be examined and corroborated with all involved in the patient's care.

A team approach is ideal. The team can consist of as few as two people which should be the physician and a nurse educated in either chemical abuse or pain management. Additional members may be a social worker, psychologist, clinical psychiatric nurse and/or substance abuse specialist. There should only be one person responsible for prescribing the narcotics so that no additional medications are ordered. Team meetings should be held to evaluate and revise the overall plan of care. Any changes in the treatment should be made known to the patient. Nursing may need to have a separate meeting to allow other staff members to vocalize any disagreements.

Realistic goals need to be set. The existence and severity of pain cannot be proven. Thus, acceptance and respect of the pain report is vital despite the fear of being duped. If you are duped, you have performed your professional responsibility. The patient _failed_ to be responsible. Rehabilitation from addiction is not appropriate when there is an acute medical problem such as pain or when it is not the patient's goal. Failure to treat pain can result in inappropriate behavior on the part of the patient and loss in confidence in the caregivers. The patient may feel that the staff is implying that he or she is lying. This can result in increased anxiety and hostility.

In assessing the patient's pain, conduct a thorough assessment. Treat any underlying causes that are amenable to standard treatments such as radiotherapy, chemotherapy, antibiotics, antifungal, and antiviral, etc. The patient needs to know that their report of pain is being taken seriously. After the assessment, changes in medication when appropriate should be accomplished. The patient may engage in normal behavior such as acting happy or laughing. This is not drug euphoria but the natural feeling of being pain free. It is important to minimize loss of control by the patient. One should try working with the patient to establish analgesic choices, doses and times. Pain and anxiety may accompany the acute pain condition and further decrease the ability to exercise control over behavior.

Sometimes it will be necessary to draw up a contract with mutually agreeable goals and expected behaviors by both the patient and the caregivers. It may be necessary to limit the amount of time the patient receives the narcotic. If the patient uses the prescribed amount of medication in a shorter period of time, then shorten the time span between visits and assess the need for a stronger dose. It is possible that the patient may not be using the medication but some family member may have gained access to the drug. All possibilities should be considered. If the contract is seriously violated, careful consideration must be given to what will be done. Other personality disorders often co-exist in substance abusers. If necessary, psychiatric consultation should be sought.

The health care professional should always keep in mind that a substance abuser can easily gain access to illegal drugs but if adequate pain relief is provided this can be avoided.

References

1. Porter J, Jick H. Addiction care in patients treated with narcotics. New Eng J Med 1980; 302, 123.

2. Angarola R. The war on drugs versus the war on cancer pain. Am J Hospice Pall Care November/December 1991; p 12-18.

3. World Health Organization (WHO) Analgesic Ladder 1990; Clinical Practice Guideline, No. 9, p. 41-45.

4. Gonzales GR, Coyle N. Treatment of cancer pain in a former opioid abuser: Fears of the patient and staff and their influence on care. J Pain Sympt Manag 1992; 7:246-249.

5. McCaffery M, Vourakis C. Assessment and relief of pain in chemically dependent patients. Orthopaedic Nursing Mar/Apr 1992; p 13-26.

6. Payne RM. Pain in the drug abuser. In: Foley KM, Payne RM. (Eds) Current therapy of pain. Philadelphia, B.C. Decker Inc. 1989; pp 46-54.

FATIGUE
Charles Kyriannis

Fatigue or asthenia refers to the sign or symptom of nonspecific generalized dysfunction. It differs from weakness which technically refers to specific muscle dysfunction. A patient often uses these terms interchangeably and simply states to the physician, "I feel weak," while actually referring to the fatigued state. It takes an astute clinician to determine its cause and offer appropriate treatment.

Fatigue has only recently been listed as an item on a checklist of symptoms in cancer patients and is being appreciated as a "multidimensional concept."[1] Different modes of expression include: physical, cognitive, activity level, motivation, and acute or chronic manifestation of these parameters. Even after fatigue has been defined and identified, the greater challenge is its measurement. Various forms of checklists and investigational instruments of varying degrees of intricacy have been devised for this purpose. Noted standards include:

> Symptom Distress Scale[2]
> Symptom Profile[3]
> Rotterdam Symptom Check List[4]
> Profile of Mood States[5]

All of these attempt to assess the chief complaint of fatigue.

In one large study of symptoms in advanced cancer patients, fatigue was the second most common complaint, pain being first. The study involved 305 patients with cancer diagnoses ranging from head and neck, breast, cervix, and lung to bone, and soft tissue. An average of 97.8% (70-100%) listed fatigue as one of their most frequent complaints.[6] In another study, 70% of patients reported fatigue - either chronic or fatigue during radiotherapy and chemotherapy.[3] Coyle et al. reported that fatigue was volunteered by 58% and 52% of patients four weeks and one week prior to death.[7]

In the last weeks of life fatigue is part of the terminal phase of illness. However, during that interim period when the patient's cancer is not causing severe symptoms, there are "nonspecific" parameters that can be followed. These reflect a patient's daily routine. Some examples include: appetite; motivation to participate in physical therapy; motivation to participate in recreational activities and the responsiveness of the patient to family and staff.

Specific physician interventions should be to assure an adequate caloric intake, correct electrolyte abnormalities, monitor adequate pain control without over sedation, and carefully evaluate for intravenous supplementation to maintain hydration.

There are many primary and secondary causes of fatigue including anemia, hypoxia, paraneoplastic syndromes, associated non cancer conditions, hypovolemia, electrolytes and metabolic disorders, drug induced causes, malnutrition, and depression.

Anemia

Anemia in this specific group of patients with advanced cancer is common. Often the drop in blood count is gradual and even if compensated for, this can cause profound fatigue. The anemia may be due to replacement of bone marrow by tumor, bleeding, cancer therapy, and dietary deficiency. The use of blood transfusion in a patient who is not a candidate for treatment with either chemotherapy or radiation and has a limited life expectancy is controversial. (It should not be based on any number [i.e., hemoglobin or hematocrit level] but whether or not it would benefit that particular patient at that particular time.) If the patient improves even for a short period of time, enabling the patient to go home, transfusion may be indicated. The risks of transfusion would, of course, be emphasized and the decision to transfuse made jointly by the patient or family and physician. The physician may need to instruct the patient and family regarding the futility of blood transfusion in some circumstances.

Hypoxia

The causes of hypoxia are many and include pleural effusions, metastases to the lung, pulmonary emboli, atelectasis, obstructive airways, pneumonia, and heart failure. We use a finger oximeter to evaluate and quantitate the percent of oxygen saturation. Generally speaking, oxygen gives subjective relief to those patients who may feel fatigued when a pulmonary or cardiac etiology is the cause. A therapeutic trial of oxygen is often the only proper measure to follow.

Paraneoplastic Syndromes

A variety of disorders that may cause weakness and fatigue due to myopathies, endocrine disturbances, and metabolic disorders may arise from paraneoplastic syndromes. All too often the disease progression causes these syndromes to worsen over time. In selected situations, corticosteroids may be indicated.

Associated Non-Cancer Illnesses

Cardiac, pulmonary, renal, and liver failure can all contribute to fatigue. These conditions become more difficult to manage in advanced cancer patients. Dosages of medication must be adjusted, routes of administration changed to accommodate particular situations, and precautions taken to prevent iatrogenically induced complications with medications such as digitalis, theophylline, tranquilizers, blood pressure medications, anxiolytics, and of course analgesics.

Diabetes should be managed carefully because nutrition in these patients is erratic and it is often difficult to maintain daily oral or injectable medications without risk of hypoglycemia. It is prudent to err on the side of allowing somewhat higher blood sugars and not attempt to obtain "tight control."

Hypovolemia, Electrolytes and Metabolic Disorders

Corrections of hypovolemia, electrolytes and metabolic disorders common in these patients may improve the symptoms of fatigue. Complications may arise as in patients with severe ascites or fluid loss from the gastrointestinal tract, fistulae, or chronic nasogastric tube suction secondary to intestinal obstruction. These situations require diligent monitoring of clinical parameters such as body weight, blood pressure, urinary output, and electrolytes. Creatinine results can also be misleading because of decreased muscle mass. Dry mucous membranes in patients who mouth breathe can lead to errors in judging the state of hydration. We make every attempt to avoid excessive venipuncture and blood tests.

At times abnormalities such as "thyroid sick cell syndrome" are encountered. This may be more of a compensatory mechanism rather than a clinical abnormality and does not warrant treatment. Aggressive attempts at correction could result in worsening of the clinical condition.

Drug Induced Causes

Opioids that are necessary for pain control have the untoward side effects of sedation and fatigue. Patients often complain of "sleeping all the time" or "being out of control" due to the confusion these medications can cause. Families complain that this limits the "quality time" they wish to spend with the patient at this crucial period. This may also interfere with the patient's activity. The art of achieving good pain control, while minimizing side effects, is a challenge to even the most experienced physician. The point to be emphasized is that opioid usage should be reevaluated often and adjustment in medications made based on the patients' complaints.

Diuretics must be used judiciously for controlling edema or ascites. Aggressive therapy can lead to hypotension and electrolyte abnormalities. Diuretics can induce hypokalemia but potassium sparing diuretics can also be hazardous in causing hyperkalemia. Beta blockers are known to cause fatigue. All medications in terminally ill patients should be carefully monitored and reevaluated when investigating a patient with a chief complaint of fatigue.

Malnutrition and depression are also important contributing factors to fatigue. A more detailed discussion may be found in chapters I,11 and IV,3.

Fatigue should not necessarily be accepted as an untreatable symptom in the cancer patient. Nothing replaces careful evaluation and reevaluation when caring for these patients. In assessing the abnormalities that contribute to the symptom of fatigue it is important to respect the compensatory mechanisms that may be at play. Overly zealous attempts to treat symptoms can worsen instead of improve a particular clinical situation.

References

1. Smets EM, Garssen B, Schuster-Uitterhoeve AL, et al. Fatigue in cancer patients. Br J Cancer Aug 1993; 68: pp 220-24.

2. McCorkle R, Quint-Benoliel J. Symptom distress, current concerns and mood disturbance after diagnosis of life-threatening disease. Soc Sci Med 1983;7:pp 431-38.

3. King KB, Nail LM, Kreamer K, et al. Patients' description of the experience of receiving radiation therapy. Onc Nurs Forum 1985;12:pp 55-61.

4. DeHaes JCJM, van Knippenberg FCE, Neijt JP. Measuring psychological and physical distress in cancer patients: structure and application of the Rotterdam Symptom Checklist. Br J Cancer 1990; 62: pp 1034-38.

5. Spiegel D, Bloom JR, Yalom I. Group support for patients with metastatic cancer. A randomized prospective out-come study. Arch Gen Psych 1981;38: pp 527-533.

6. Sebastian P, Varghese C, Sankaranarayanan R, et al. Evaluation of symptomatology in planning palliative care. Palliat Med 1993;7: pp 27-34.

7. Coyle N, Adelhardt J, Foley KM, Portenoy RK. J Pain Sympt Manag 1990;5: pp 83-93.

DYSPNEA I
Michael J. Brescia

Of all the symptoms associated with advanced cancer, dyspnea is probably the most difficult to manage. It produces unacceptable suffering and is often the most poorly controlled. Some patients may present with such severe symptomatology that they offer a rational and emotional assent for assisted suicide, intensified by family members who also wish to see an end to the suffering. We have witnessed countless cases of death associated with severe air hunger. Patients suffer with tachypnea and cyanosis, with no hope of relief. Hence, the dyspneic patient must be aggressively treated.

Dyspnea, by definition, is the feeling that one cannot exert him or herself any further. Although it is a protective mechanism to prevent human beings from over exertion, the obvious outcome diminishes quality of life. A majority of patients in the last six weeks of life suffer a form of dyspnea and only a small percent experience an alleviation of symptoms.

Dyspnea is most commonly seen in breast, lung, prostate, and colon cancers. The major causes of dyspnea include:

- Bronchial pneumonia
- Carcinomatous lymphangitis
- Superior vena cava syndrome
- Neoplastic replacement of the lung
- Tracheo-esophageal fistula
- Vocal cord paralysis
- Ascites
- Diaphragmatic paresis, unilateral and bilateral
- Cardiomyopathy
- Embolism
- Pericardial effusion.

Treatment Protocols

Bronchial pneumonia is treated with appropriate supportive measures including positioning and promotion of cough along with antibiotics when indicated. It is critical to dispel the concept of pneumonia as being the companion of the aged and infirm. Often a protracted pneumonia with concurrent dyspnea can be rapidly controlled with antibiotics.

Carcinomatous lymphangitis is extremely disabling. Wherever possible, susceptible tumors should be treated with chemotherapy, radiotherapy and/or large doses of steroids.

The superior vena caval syndrome can respond to both chemotherapy and radiotherapy. It should be pretreated with large doses of steroids.

Neoplastic replacement of the lung represents a significant challenge for therapy. In general, such patients require large doses of opioids for control of symptoms. Rarely is chemotherapy indicated.

Tracheo-esophageal fistulae in a palliative setting are usually seen after esophageal stents have been inserted. Their success is limited and temporary. Direct surgical procedures are generally not indicated or possible. Bypassing the fistula with a gastrostomy can minimize aspiration pneumonia and the accompanying dyspnea. Vocal cord paralysis eventually progresses to stenosis and upper airway obstruction. Permanent tracheostomy provides a large measure of relief.

In patients with ascites, one of the most neglected and effective treatments is paracentesis. Even the removal of two liters of fluid provides the immediate relief of dyspnea.

Small multiple emboli may be treated with anticoagulants thus removing the etiologic focus and reducing the degree of dyspnea. If an acute, massive pulmonary embolus occurs resulting in an agonal event, therapy with opioids without anticoagulation is indicated.

Pericardial effusions are almost always associated with severe dyspnea and should be treated with pericardiocentesis and/or formation of a pericardial window. Where the pathology of the tumor offers a reasonable chance of palliation, external radiation therapy and chemotherapy may be indicated.

Drug Therapy

The drugs most frequently administered in the symptomatic treatment of patients include theophylline, prostaglandin inhibitors, benzodiazepines, lidocaine via nebulizer for intractable cough, and finally, opioid therapy.

In controlling dyspnea which can not be managed by any other measure, opioids are the drugs of choice. Opioids have multiple pharmacologic effects including decreasing oxygen consumption, and diminishing ventilatory response to hypoxia and hypercapnia. As the CO_2 level rises, dyspnea dramatically abates. At levels of PCO_2 of 75 mm, dyspnea significantly decreases possibly due to the release of endorphins. Exogenous opioids can quickly initiate endorphin effect.

Opioid receptors are present in the respiratory tree and it is possible that blockage of these receptors is what contributes to the relief of breathlessness. Nebulization of opioids has been studied in several centers with mixed conclusions of efficacy. The dosing frequency and outcome measurements have not been standardized.

Case Examples

The following patient profiles illustrate suffering from advanced pulmonary insufficiency in which severe dyspnea was relieved.

Patient #1　　52 Y/O with cancer of the lower trachea and carina, status post-chemotherapy and radiotherapy and stent failure. There was intractable dyspnea and psychological, familial and staff reactions due to unrelenting stridor.

Patient #2　　27 Y/O with disseminated Kaposi's sarcoma. There was neoplastic replacement of both lungs with complete therapeutic failure. There had been intractable dyspnea for two weeks.

Patient #3　　72 Y/O physician with tracheo-esophageal fistula and severe intractable dyspnea with unreachable retained secretions. Therapeutic failure caused the patient to plead for euthanasia.

In the foregoing three patients, pain was never an issue. All the suffering was caused by pulmonary failure and intractable complications resulting in severe permanent breathlessness. A consolidated approach and goal of therapy in each case was to relieve the dyspnea and thereby reduce an unacceptable level of suffering. This included the use of IV bolus morphine (5-10 mg IV) every 15 minutes until the patient no longer experienced the sensation of dyspnea. This might require three to four cycles. When the patient became comfortable, a maintenance dose of either IV morphine continuously administered or bolus morphine given subcutaneously was administered. This maintained a clinically satisfactory result. Failure to control the dyspnea in these patients would have caused protracted suffering.

General supportive measures include a cool room, O_2 via a mask at 8-10L/min to produce a comfortable effect from the circulation of a soft breeze across the nares and face, frequent brief periods of suctioning where applicable, and proper positioning in bed or chair.

Use of restraints to control an anxious patient is considered a failure in medical therapy. During the control phase of dyspnea, staff, families, friends or volunteers should provide a human presence at the bedside gently restraining a frightened or confused patient. The sight of limb restraints on a struggling patient is neither morally nor professionally acceptable.

Dyspnea challenges the mind and spirit of all who labor with compromised patients.

DYSPNEA II - SPECIAL CONSIDERATIONS: MALIGNANT PLEURAL EFFUSIONS; PULSE OXIMETRY
Joseph Casino

Malignant Pleural Effusions

Patients with malignant pleural effusions generally have a very poor prognosis with a survival of only 3 - 16 months. The primary diagnosis influences survival. Patients with effusions secondary to lung cancer usually have a shorter survival than those patients with breast cancer. A classical study of 30 years ago demonstrated a 1 - 2 months survival in patients who meet the criteria of pleural fluid pH <7.3 and glucose <60mg/dl.[1] These findings remain valid today.

The presence of an effusion does not always indicate incurability. The effusion may be paramalignant and not directly involve the pleura or may be related to an obstructing bronchial lesion with atelectasis, pneumonia or some concurrent illness such as congestive heart failure.

Some of the mechanisms that can cause pleural effusion in the presence of malignant disease are:[2]

> Pleural metastases with increased permeability
>   or obstruction of pleural lymphatic vessels
> Mediastinal lymph node involvement with decreased
>   pleural lymphatic drainage
> Bronchial obstruction causing decreased pleural pressures
> Postobstructive pneumonitis
> Thoracic duct interruption
> Pericardial invasion
> Hypoproteinemia
> Pulmonary embolism
> Postradiation therapy.

In another early study, lung cancer was the most common cause of malignant pleural effusions and accounts for approximately 30% of all effusions. Other tumors that cause malignant effusions are breast (25%), lymphoma (20%), ovarian carcinoma (6%) and sarcomas, especially melanoma (3%). The primary tumor is never identified in 6% of patients.[3]

Treatment

If the patient is asymptomatic, observation may be reasonable, but inevitably the effusion will progress and become symptomatic.

Serial therapeutic thoracenteses with removal of fluid is useful if the fluid does not re-accumulate rapidly. These procedures can be performed on an outpatient basis and this may allow time for a patient to undergo chemotherapy. Serial thoracenteses may also avoid the need for invasive thoracostomy tube drainage with instillation of sclerosing agents.

Thoracostomy tube drainage alone is not recommended because it rarely results in adequate pleural abrasion and sclerosis which are necessary to control the effusion.

Some therapists advocate the use of serial intrapleural injections of corynebacterium parvum or chemical agents. However, the majority of pulmonologists generally choose thoracostomy tube insertion and drainage of the effusions and when the fluid efflux falls to <150cc/day, instillation of a sclerosing agent. In a properly selected population this can achieve control of effusions in 80 - 90% of patients.

The available chemical agents which have demonstrated adequate sclerosing properties include minocycline and doxycycline (since tetracycline is no longer commercially available.) Bleomycin has been shown to have high efficacy but is limited by its high cost and potential for systemic side effects. Installation of talc in a preparation of a sterile slurry or talc poudrage via thoracoscopy can also be highly effective. Chemical pleurodesis commonly fails if the lung is not adequately re-expanded. Pleural abrasion with pleurectomy is nearly 100% effective and is now performed under video assisted thoracoscopic surgery (VATS.)

Systemic chemotherapy may also be of value even when cure is not possible. On the other hand, radiation therapy to the corresponding hemithorax is generally contraindicated since it may worsen symptoms if radiation pneumonitis should occur. A synopsis of malignant pleural effusions was recently reported in the *American Journal of Hospice and Palliative Care*.[3]

Pulse oximetry and management of the patient with dyspnea

Dyspnea is always a distressing symptom but particularly in the population of patients with terminal illness. Patients with advanced disease, either cardiopulmonary or malignant may experience breathlessness secondary to an age related decline in respiratory function and concomitant cardiopulmonary illness. This may limit activity, function, and consequently quality of life.

A universally accepted definition of dyspnea does not exist. The roots of dyspnea, dys(disordered) and pnea(breathing), help put the definition into perspective.

Increasing the fractional inspired oxygen concentration (F_iO_2) causes pulmonary and vascular resistance to fall with subsequent improvement in dyspnea. Oxygen administration is also relatively innocuous in the palliative care population although we must acknowledge the possibility of depression of respiratory drive in patients with altered chemotherapy and oxygen receptor response to hypercapnia/hypoxemia. The basis for administration of oxygen is founded on the physiology of gas exchange and oxygen transport to tissues. Arterial oxygen concentration (P_aO_2) is determined by the fractional inspired oxygen concentration (F_iO_2), ventilation/perfusion matching (V/Q), and diffusion of gases across the alveolar-capillary basement membrane. Oxygen is the only proven therapy which will prolong life in the patient with advanced chronic obstructive pulmonary disease. Oxygen therapy is important to reverse life threatening hypoxemia, but an increase in arterial carbon dioxide concentration (P_aCO_2) and a fall in pH suggest hypoventilation. Many spirited discussions have taken place in the literature on whether excessive oxygen administration in patients with chronic CO_2 retention is detrimental. On balance, adequate oxygen should be administered to prevent hypoxemia and ultimately dyspnea. Concomitant administration of morphine will also serve in decreasing air hunger.

In the palliative care population arterial blood gases are infrequently utilized primarily because of the discomfort of arterial punctures. It is with this goal in mind that pulse oximetry represents an advantage when monitoring oxygen saturation noninvasively. Pulse oximetry is the indirect measurement of oxygen saturation by analyzing the pulsatile change in light transmission through living tissue, understanding that such a change in light transmission would be due to a change in their intervening blood volume. The absorption of light by tissue, bone, skin, pigments and venous blood are eliminated from consideration. The Oximeter calculates the ratio of the pulse added absorbance at different wave lengths of light employed. The hemoglobin saturation is calculated by an empirical algorithm. The ratio of measured absorbencies is converted to a specific saturation value based on results of previous data in normal persons in whom the oximeter was calibrated against measurements of absolute arterial oxygen saturation. There are limitations and pitfalls of following oxygen saturations by pulse oximetry. First and foremost hemoglobin saturation increases little as the arterial oxygen concentration (P_aO_2) increases above 60 mmHg and exhibits almost no change if oxygen saturation exceeds 100%. Therefore, if the P_aO_2 is approximately 170 with supplemental oxygen in place there is a possibility of an adverse physiologic trend occurring. The clinician may be entirely unaware of this because the oxygen saturation would remain 100% despite a decrease in P_aO_2 from 170 to 80 mmHg. Another potential pitfall is based on the knowledge that even a relatively small degree of inaccuracy in oxygen saturation measurements can have a large impact on assumed corresponding arterial oxygen concentration. There is an accepted 95% confidence level on non-invasive oximetry which still represents a potential error of 3-5%. Therefore, a measured saturation of 95% ± 4% (91-99%) could be associated with a P_aO_2 value from 60 mmHg 91% to 160 mmHg 99% saturation.

If a significant concentration of carboxyhemoglobin or methemoglobin is present, oximeters are unable to distinguish them from oxyhemoglobin and thus will be reflected as a falsely elevated oxygen saturation. Motion and dislodgement of the probe in agitated patients also limits its utility and effectiveness. Skin pigmentation does not effect oximetry since only the pulse added change in absorption is considered. Nail polish needs to be removed because any absorption of light by the polish could render a signal weak and inaccurate. Adequate tissue perfusion pressure is required so that the oximeter can sense a pulse with oxygen saturation below 65% oximetry is less reliable.

Oximetry can provide adequate saturation readings in patients with leukemia or severe leucocytosis.

Oximetry also allows the titration of oxygen to an acceptable flow rate in liters/min. Despite its limitations, pulse oximetry represents a noninvasive method of assessing oxygen saturation, useful in the palliative care population, when patient comfort is the primary goal. In addition, it is a means of documenting the need for long term oxygen therapy as determined by Medicare and most insurance carriers.

References

1. Spriggs AI, Boddington MM. The cytology of effusions. New York: Grune & Stratton 1968, 2nd ed.

2. Light RW. Pleural diseases. Philadelphia: Lea & Febiger, 1990, 2nd ed., p 99.

3. Anderson CB, Philpott GW, Ferguson TB. The treatment of malignant pleural effusions. Cancer 1974;33:pp 916-922.

4. Rousseau P. Current concepts in pain management - malignant pleural effusions: A brief synopsis. Am J Hospice & Pall Care 1997;14:pp 302-304.

GASTROINTESTINAL MALIGNANT OBSTRUCTION
Michael J. Brescia

Gastrointestinal obstruction (GI) is usually associated with great suffering with symptomatology that is particularly distressing to the patient. It always requires aggressive treatment. Physician intervention should be rigorous and definitive with a view toward making a diagnosis as soon as possible to produce adequate palliation and relief of symptoms.

The most common malignancies causing gastrointestinal obstruction include ovary, rectum, colon, caecum, stomach, endometrium, prostate, and bladder in descending order. In the gastrointestinal tract, the most common sites of early obstruction include the gastroduodenal region, the small bowel, and the colon, especially at the splenic flexure. Although the esophagus frequently obstructs, it will not be discussed in this section.

Types of Bowel Obstruction

Clinicians are most familiar with direct invasive metastatic disease causing GI obstruction.

Intraluminal tumors, especially of the right colon, are usually polypoid lesions which lead to obstruction and can present with acute dilatation proximal to the obstructing lesion. Fecal impaction may also develop and accelerate obstruction.

Intramural obstruction involves the musculature of the gut.

Extramural tumors produce extrinsic compression and are located in the omentum and mesentery. Sites of GI obstruction may be multiple.

Motility dysfunction may be a source obstruction due to impaired or destroyed innervation of parts of the GI tract. This commonly occurs in patients with ovarian tumors. The pathophysiology usually involves a metastatic mesenteric lesion due to a large tumor having destroyed a nerve adjacent to a segment of gut.

Inflammatory obstruction resulting from local non-specific reactive edema in tumors can respond to anti-inflammatory therapy.

Symptoms

The most common symptoms in gastrointestinal obstruction include: abdominal distention; flatulence; ascites; colicky abdominal pain; pain at the site of the metastasis; constipation and/or diarrhea; nausea and vomiting; tenesmus; retro-cardiac pain;

belching, drooling; hiccups and dysphagia. These symptoms must be aggressively addressed and are usually relieved with the correction of the obstruction.

At Calvary Hospital, surgical intervention is usually not an option because of multiple metastatic deposits and motility dysfunction. However, surgery may be considered if relief of the obstruction will result in extending a reasonable period of comfortable life. Before ruling out surgical intervention one must be certain that the obstruction is not of benign origin which may have been the result of prior surgery or radiotherapy.

Definitive Therapy for Gastrointestinal Obstruction

Surgery to relieve gastric outlet obstruction should be a consideration, if this is the first episode of obstruction and there is only one primary site delineated. Far advanced carcinoma can produce multiple sites of obstruction and therefore, yield a poor chance of surgical improvement.

If there are local additional measures to be considered local, single masses radiotherapy or chemotherapy should be considered in certain select tumors, for example, lymphomas.

Immediate measures should be taken to determine the site of the obstruction. Flat plates supine and uprights are taken to search for localized areas of gut dilatation. Absorbable contrast media for upper GI delineation of the obstructive site can also be utilized. Endoscopy, including gastroscopy and sigmocolonoscopy, may be indicated.

Venting Obstructed Gut

Excess intestinal volume must be drained. This can be done successfully with intubation and suction. IV fluids are administered as necessary. The best way to reduce intestinal volume is venting. The obstructed area with its accumulating fluid can be vented outside the body via gastrostomy, colostomy, jejunostomy, and cecostomy. This may be facilitated with the use of a suction pump.

Contributory Factors

When possible, treat any contributory factors. Gastroparesis can be caused by diminished peristalsis due to diminished gut musculature, innervation, malnutrition, low residue diet, or low oral fluid volume. This may also be induced by drugs, especially opioids, diabetes, advanced AIDS, and general cachexia. Prokinetic agents can be useful.

A search for intestinal infection which can produce gut dilatation, such as Clostridia Difficile may respond to antibiotic therapy.

General Measures and Considerations

Constipation and fecal impaction must be vigorously treated but preferably prevented. Daily enemas can relieve obstruction due to feces. Oral medication can also be beneficial when the patient is able to swallow. A frequent cause of GI obstruction is due to overly aggressive therapy for diarrhea. The use of loperamide (Immodium) and especially atropine diphenoxylate (Lomotil) must be monitored carefully.

History and physical assessment is crucial. Palpable masses and organs must be evaluated. Ascites frequently will confirm a diagnosis of advanced GI malignancy. The persistence, color, and volume of vomitus may indicate an upper GI obstruction. The more frequent and the greater the volume of the vomitus, the more likely that a high GI obstruction is present.

Nausea and Vomiting

Intubation and drainage for upper GI malignancies provide rapid decline of nausea and vomiting in resistant symptoms due to a high GI obstruction. Venting the fluid can produce significant palliation rapidly and reduce the level of suffering. When drainage volume falls suction may temporarily be discontinued. Occasionally nausea and vomiting may not recur even after tube drainage has been discontinued. The indications for a venting gastrostomy include high to mid-high small bowel obstruction. In a home care environment this can be a valuable adjunct to therapy.

Hiccoughs

Hiccoughs is a debilitating and tenacious symptom that can persist unremittingly for weeks. Upon admission, patients often have persistent hiccoughs as a major complaint. Hiccoughs may sometimes be controlled with simple decompression of the stomach. One should also consider steroids, compazine, and more recently, baclofin which decreases the severity and amplitude of the diaphragmatic motion. If a patient has ascites, paracentesis can quickly relieve hiccoughs.

Tenesmus

Tenesmus is treated with antispasmodics or with a catheter inserted into the rectum and a lidocaine - saline drip which can anesthetize the mucosal surface.

Abdominal Distension

A venting procedure such as, gastrostomy, jejunostomy or colostomy should be considered for abdominal distention which is persistent and unremitting. Infections and fecal obstruction are treated. The site of a discreet obstruction is identified where possible.

Conclusion

Most of the symptoms in malignant gastrointestinal obstruction are rapidly relieved by surgical intervention when this is appropriate in view of the patient's overall prognosis. Venting the obstructing gut either surgically or by tube drainage is also helpful.

In the presence of ascites paracentesis can produce instant relief of symptoms even when as little as one liter of fluid is successfully drained. In rare instances and with responsive tumors, radiotherapy and chemotherapy may produce palliation.

Unless the obstructive symptoms are physiologic or metabolic, drug therapy alone is disappointing and not successful.

Of interest in our experience at Calvary Hospital, the longest lived patients with GI obstruction are those that have developed fistulae relieving the obstruction. Carcinomas of the colon and ovary may cause venting via the vagina and although aesthetically undesirable, can lead to a prolongation of life. No studies have been done to evaluate the quality of life after spontaneous fistulous venting.

The use of IV fluids and electrolyte replacement should be administered carefully so that the volume of gastrointestinal secretions are not increased by over hydration.

It is important to recognize that after the diagnosis of malignant GI obstruction is made the average life span is 29 days. Therefore, therapy should take this into consideration.

NAUSEA AND VOMITING
Rekha Mehta

Nausea and vomiting are common distressing complaints in palliative medicine and oncology practice. In one of the earliest studies of 1,596, 62% of terminally ill cancer patients reported nausea or vomiting at some time during the last six weeks of life.[1]

Stimuli and neural pathways are common for both nausea and vomiting. Nausea is more akin to a psychic phenomenon or an unpleasant sensation felt by the patient. It may not always evolve into an act of vomiting. Retching causes spasmodic contractions of the same group of muscles without production of vomitus. It is also known as dry heaves since gastric contents are not brought up. During retching the glottis is closed and there is rapid decrease in intrathoracic pressure and increase in the intra-abdominal pressure. The act of vomiting on the other hand, is associated with increase in the intrathoracic as well as intra-abdominal pressure. The diaphragm muscles are involved. This is accompanied by a forceful ejection of gastric contents with regurgitation. Gastric contents are brought up without contractions of the above group of muscles and autonomic activity is not involved. When regurgitated food is swallowed back and chewed, it is called rumination.[2]

Hypersalivation may accompany nausea. Retching may be associated with atrial tachycardia and vomiting may be accompanied by bradycardia. Very rarely defecation may accompany vomiting.

Physiology

The vomiting center is located in the reticular formation of the medulla. Direct electrical stimulation of this area is followed by vomiting. It can also be stimulated by visceral afferent impulses from the gastrointestinal tract, pharynx, heart, peritoneum, mesentery, and bile ducts.[3] The chemoreceptor trigger zone (CTZ) is located in the floor of the fourth ventricle in the area postrema. CTZ does not respond to electrical stimuli but responds to chemical stimuli in the circulation. The dopamine receptors in CTZ play a role in mediating vomiting. Drugs, uremia, hypoxia, labyrinthine stimulation, diabetic ketoacidosis, and radiation stimulate CTZ to induce vomiting.

Causes of Nausea and Vomiting

The list of causes for nausea and vomiting is long. Table 1 lists the most likely encountered in palliative medicine. There may be multiple contributing factors in one individual. (See Table 1)

Table 1

Oropharyngeal	Fungating head and neck tumors Herpetic infection Candida infection

Gastrointestinal	a) Esophageal:
	    Obstructing cancer
	    Achalasia
	    Gastric reflux
	
	b) Gastric:
	    Outlet obstruction due to tumor
	    Motility disorder due to:
	        - Ascites
	        - Drugs (Morphine, anticholinergics)
	        - Extrinsic pressure due to large tumor mass (squashed stomach syndrome)
	
	c) Intestinal
	    Obstruction
	    Pseudo-obstruction
	    Paralytic ileus

Visceral Pain:	Renal, biliary, intestinal colic Intestinal ischemia Stretched liver capsule due to tumor Pancreatitis Myocardial infarction
Neurological:	Increased intracranial tension due to metastasis
Vestibular	Middle ear infection, viral neuronitis, cerebellopontine tumor
Drugs	Chemotherapy, radiation therapy, estrogen, analgesics (opiod and nonopioids)
Metabolic	Uremia, Addisons disease, hypercalcemia

Psychogenic

                    Conditioned reflexes - offensive odors, sights
                    Anxiety
                    Depression

Generally, with regurgitation small amounts of clear mucoid secretions are brought up. It is associated with obstructing nasopharyngeal tumors and esophageal tumors. The gastric outlet obstruction produces large volume vomitus of undigested food. The act of vomiting may cause petechiae over the face and upper neck area. A violent retching may cause a mucosal tear at the gastroesophageal junction and cause bleeding. Recurrent vomiting causes increase in fluid loss, dehydration, sodium (Na) and potassium (K) depletion, and metabolic alkalosis. The abdominal exam is important to check for intestinal obstruction, organomegaly or ascites. Occasionally upright abdominal films are necessary to differentiate between intestinal obstruction and paralytic ileus.

Treatment

Intravenous fluids with Na and K repletion may become necessary. In patients with intestinal obstruction or gastric outlet obstruction, insertion of a nasogastric tube may provide tremendous relief. This intervention alone, when connected to intermittent suction, may sufficiently alleviate vomiting. It is not uncommon for a terminally ill patient to request "no tubes." In such cases, it is advisable to curtail oral intake and prescribe medications for nausea and vomiting. Some patients may express a strong desire to receive food by mouth. After careful evaluation of the patient, fluids are permissible even while a nasogastric tube is connected to intermittent suction.

Medical treatment of nausea and vomiting may include sedation, cholinergic antagonism, H_1 receptor blockade, dopamine antagonism or serotonin 5-hydroxytryptamine (5HT) blockade. Generally, antihistamine drugs of H_1 type like meclizine and cyclizine are used in vomiting episodes due to motion sickness or labyrinthine stimulation. Anticholinergic drugs like scopolamine can also be used in motion sickness. When symptoms are primarily due to regurgitation or increased salivary secretions with obstructing pharyngeal or esophageal tumors, atropine 0.2 - 0.4 mg subcutaneously or intramuscularly may be useful. Amitriptyline can also be used as an adjunct by drying out the oral secretions. For nausea, phenothiazines, such as, perphenazine, prochlorperazine, chlorpromazine, and promethazine are most commonly prescribed in the palliative setting. Haloperidol can be useful in controlling vomiting induced by drugs. Haloperidol actually acts by blocking dopamine action on CTZ. We have also used promethazine drip intravenously. Prokinetic agents like metoclopramide act on CTZ by blocking dopamine receptors. Metoclopramide is very useful in severe reflux disease, gastric stasis, gastroparesis, pseudo-obstruction, and ileus. A dose of up to 80 mg is tolerated, but incidence of side effects escalates with doses above 40 mg. Adverse reactions may occur in 20% of the cases and include drowsiness, akathisia, tremor, dystonic reaction, and anxiety. Extrapyramidal

Parkinsonian reactions resolve with withdrawal of the drug. Occasionally breast enlargement, galactorrhea or menstrual irregularity may be seen due to prolactin release.[4] Domperidone and cisapride are other prokinetic agents.

Tetrahydrocannabinol (THC), the active ingredient of marijuana is also effective in chemotherapy induced nausea and vomiting.[5] Oral synthetic cannabinoid (Nabilone) is used in 1-2 mg doses every 8 hours. Levonantroidol can be used parenterally or orally. The toxicity at higher doses cause urinary retention. Drowsiness, hypotension, tachycardia, dry mouth, hallucinations, dysphoria, and even psychosis may be seen. Usage has decreased with the availability of other choices. (See Pharmacy section of this book.)

Steroids have unexplained antiemetic activity and are useful in combination with phenothiazines or metoclopramide. The activity is probably related to an antiprostaglandin effect. They are primarily used in patients with brain tumors due to increased intracranial pressure.

Ondansetron, a selective 5 - hydroxytryptamine ($5\text{-}HT_3$) antagonist, a newer antiemetic can be used intravenously or orally. It has rapid onset of action and it is well tolerated.[6] It is perhaps more effective than metoclopramide[7] and even provides relief from cholestasis induced pruritus.[8] Extrapyramidal reactions like opisthotonos, stiffness, involuntary head jerking, and akathisia, although rare, have been reported.[9] The usefulness of this drug at present is limited by its cost.

In summary, in the palliative setting the etiology of nausea and vomiting should be quickly established with history and physical exam. The medications should be kept simple and the easiest route of administration individually determined. If the patient refuses injections or chooses oral or rectal suppositories, they should be tried. On the other hand if IV access is feasible then IV drugs may be preferred. (See the Pharmacy section of this book for medications used at Calvary Hospital.)

References

1. Reuben DB, Mor V. Nausea and vomiting in terminal cancer patients. Arch Intern Med 1986; 146: pp 2021-2023.

2. Hanson JS, McCallum RW. The diagnosis and management of nausea and vomiting: a review. Am J. Gastro 1985; 80: pp 210-218.

3. Borison HL, Wang SC. Physiology and pharmacology of vomiting. Pharmacol Rev 1953; 5: pp 193-230.

4. Albibi R, McCallum RW. Metoclopramide: pharmacology and clinical application. Ann Int Med 1983;98: pp 86-95.

5. Vincent BJ, McQuiston DJ, Einhorn LH, et al. Review of cannabinoids and their antiemetic effectiveness. Drugs 1983; 25 (Suppl 1) pp 52-62.

6. Currow DC, Coughlan M, Fardell B, et al. Use of ondansetron in palliative medicine. J Pain Symptom Manag 1997;13: pp 302-307.

7. DeMulder PH, Seyraeve C, Vermorken JB, et al. Ondansetron compared with high dose metoclopramide in prophylaxis of acute and delayed cisplatin-induced nausea and vomiting; a multicenter, randomized double-blind, crossover study. Ann Int Med 1990; 113: pp 834-840.

8. Schworer H, Hartmann H, Ramadon G. Relief of cholestatic pruritis by a novel class of drugs: $5HT_3$ receptor antagonists: effectiveness of ondansetron. Pain 1995; 61: pp 33-37.

9. Halperin JR, Murphy B. Extrapyramidal reaction to ondansetron. Cancer 1992;69: p 1275.

SEIZURES
Antonios Vlantis

It is estimated that 1% of the patients with disseminated cancer or 20-50% of all patients with brain tumors (primary or metastatic) experience seizures. Patients with CNS infections (after bone marrow transplantation), as well as patients with leptomeningeal metastases and other neurologic complications of cancer, are prone to seizures. Seizures are more commonly experienced in patients with multiple metastases, melanoma, in patients with combined brain and leptomeningeal metastases, and in those with multiple myeloma. Seizures are either focal motor, beginning with a chronic jerking of the face or of one extremity, or may manifest to involve the other extremity of the same size, or progress to a grand mal seizure. Infrequently seizures do progress to status epilepticus.

Causes

Causes of seizures in patients with cancer are listed as follows:

Metastatic CNS cancers, both parenchymal and leptomeningeal;

Primary brain tumors - gliomas, meningiomas;

Metabolic disturbances - hyponatremia (SIADH), hypoxia, hypocalcemia and hypomagnesemia, hepatic encephalopathy, uremia;

Infections - bacterial (listeria monocyte genes), viral (cytomegalovirus - herpes), parasites (toxoplasma gandii), fungal (cryptococcus, Aspergillus);

Treatment related etiologies,

Radiation (acute-delayed),
Chemotherapy

Medications - opiates (particularly meperidine and others in the presence of renal failure), antibiotics (penicillin, imipenem-cilastatin), tricylic antidepressants, antiemetic (phenothiazines - butyrophenones), amphetamines, drug withdrawal (benzodiazepines and barbiturates.)

Differential Diagnoses

Sometimes epileptic seizures (ES) can be confused with nonepileptic seizures (NES). It is important to diagnose patients with nonepileptic seizures since they can be submitted to a variety of iatrogenic hazards due to administration of antiepileptic medications. (In addition, these patients consume important medical resources through physician and emergency department visits.)

True epileptic seizures usually have to be differentiated from psychologic disorders (like conversion disorders), cardiovascular disorders (syncope, arrhythmias), migraine syndromes, and sleep disorders. To distinguish between epileptic and nonepileptic seizures, detailed history, physical examinations, psychologic testing, and EEG findings are very important. Epileptic seizures are always accompanied by abnormal electrical activity in the brain.

Pathogenesis of seizures in primary or metastatic brain tumors

Although the precise pathogenesis of seizures due to brain tumors is unknown, it is believed that a breakdown of the blood-brain barrier and brain edema play a role. Edema fluid has a higher potassium concentration than does normal brain extracellular fluid, possibly promoting depolarization of neurons, which can lead to seizures. Tumor growth is not the only mechanism which can disrupt the blood-brain barrier and cause edema. In metastatic brain tumors, leaky neovessels within the tumor and altered normal vessels in the tissue surrounding the tumor also lead to the formation of brain edema. An increase in hydrostatic pressure can disrupt the barrier and lead to brain edema. Compression of nervous system tissue may also disrupt the barrier, possibly by interfering with venous drainage thus increasing capillary hydrostatic pressure. Radiation and chemotherapy also effect the blood-brain barrier.

Treatment

Although prophylactic anticonvulsant therapy is controversial, some physicians do use antiepileptic treatment in patients with primary or metastatic brain tumors. Calvary physicians are divided in the use of prophylactic therapy. However, since melanoma causes both, multiple parenchymal and leptomeningeal metastases, and the incidence of seizures is high (50%), most consultants do recommend prophylaxis in these patients.

The most commonly used anticonvulsant is phenytoin in a loading dose of 100 mg (or 15 - 20 mg/Kg) given in divided doses over the first 24 hours, followed by 300 - 400 mg (or 5 - 6 mg/Kg) daily. Phenytoin given intravenously can cause hypotension and should not be given more rapidly than 50 mg/min. Phenytoin is not given IM as it is painful and absorption is erratic. Phenytoin toxicity includes sedation, cognitive changes, ataxia, dysarthria and mysteyomm. Alternatives to phenytoin include sodium valporoate, carbamazepine, phenobarbital or clonazepam for the immediate treatment of seizures, diazepam in a dose of 0.25 mg/Kg IV (up to 20 mg). This should be given at a rate less than 5 mg/min. The same dose of diazepam can be used for status epilepticus, followed by phenytoin 15-20 mg/Kg IV at 50 mg/min or less. Clonazepam 1 mg IV is an alternative to intravenous diazepam or lorazepan 0.1 mg/Kg IV (< 2 mg/min) over 15 - 60 min. Phenobarbital also can be used 20 mg/Kg IV (< 100/min), over 60-120 min.

Patients requiring maintenance anticonvulsant therapy and who are unable to swallow medications, may be treated as follows: phenobarbital 100 mg IM or 400 - 600 mg daily for the water soluble preparation by continuous SC infusion, rectal diazepam or clonazepam 1-5 mg/day by continuous SC infusion. For focal seizures phenytoin or carbamazepine can be used effectively. Corticosteroids in high doses may also be used to reduce cerebral edema.

Side effects of anticonvulsants

There is little evidence supporting the superiority of one drug over another. Monotherapy is usually better than polytherapy providing that maximally tolerated doses of the single agent are used. Recent evidence suggests that almost all anticonvulsants produce drowsiness and cognitive dysfunction. Patients may tolerate one medication better than another. Carbamazepine and primidone may cause profound drowsiness and may not be tolerated if given at full doses.

The main side effect of anticonvulsants are listed as follows:

Dose related:

Dizziness - ataxia (phenytoin);
Cognitive dysfunction (all);
Diplopia (carbamazepine, phenytoin);
Myopathy (phenytoin);
Asterixis (all).

Metabolic:

Osteomalacia (phenytoin);

Elevated liver enzymes (phenytoin, carbamazepine).

Other less common toxicities:

Stevens-Johnson Syndrome (carbamazepine - phenytoin);
Vasculitis (phenytoin);
Arthritis - shoulder-hand syndrome (phenobarbital);
Stupor (valerate);
Meningitis (carbamazepine);
Agranulocytosis (carbamazepine);
Pseudolymphoma (phenytoin).

Some excellent and pertinent studies are listed in the references.

References

1. Cohen N, Straus G, Lew SR, et al. Should prophylactic anti-convulsants be administered to patients with newly-diagnosed cerebral metastases? A retrospective analysis. J Clin Oncol 1991;6:pp 1621-1624.

2. Weaver S, Forsythe P, Fulton D, et al. A prospective, randomized study of prophylactic anticonvulsants in patients with primary brain tumors or metastatic brain tumors and without prior seizures. A preliminary analysis of 67 patients (Abstract 371P). In Neurology 1995;45 (suppl 4):A263.

3. Glantz MJ, Cole BF, Friedberg MH, et al. A randomized blinded, placebo-controlled trial of divalproex sodium prophyaxis in adults with newly diagnosed brain tumors. Neurology 1996;46:p 98.

4. Batchelor TT, DeAngelis LM, Medical management of cerebral metastases. In Harsh GR (ed): Neurological Clinics 1996;7:p 435.

DELIRIUM AND DEPRESSION
Robert A. Brescia

Advanced cancer patients experience and exhibit many painful and distressing psychiatric symptoms. All too often these symptoms go unrecognized and/or untreated. Those of us working in this field are usually quite good at recognizing and treating our patients' physical symptoms and physical pain. Recognizing and treating our patients' psychiatric symptoms and psychic pain can be difficult. Nevertheless, once recognized these distressing symptoms can often be treated with measures that are relatively simple and safe. Every effort should be made to accurately diagnosis psychiatric abnormalities.

At Calvary Hospital, patients are evaluated by the psychiatrist at the request of the attending physician. Sometimes these requests are prompted by the nurse, another team member, the patient's family, or the patient. The most common symptoms which lead to psychiatric intervention are those of delirium and depression. These conditions can and do cause terrible distress. Fortunately, appropriate intervention can greatly reduce the emotional pain.

Delirium is defined as "a constellation of cognitive, behavioral and psychological abnormalities associated with a transient or permanent dysfunction of the brain." Approximately 85% of hospitalized cancer patients suffer from delirium at some point prior to death.[1] In advanced cancer there are many factors that can contribute to the development of delirium including: medications (analgesics, sedatives, steroids, etc.), infection, anemia, CNS metastasis, metabolic disorders, organ failure, and fluid-electrolyte imbalance. Symptoms of delirium include cognitive impairment, decreased alertness and awareness of the environment, reduced capacity to shift, focus and sustain attention, change in sleep-wake cycle, poor social judgment, decreased impulse control, mood disturbance, change in psychomotor behavior and paranoia, delusions and hallucinations.

Practically speaking, what we observe is often a dramatic change in the patient's mental status developing over a period of only minutes in some cases to several days in others. This "dramatic change" can present in many different ways. Some common variations are as follows:

A pleasant, engaging patient suddenly becomes angry, hostile and perhaps even threatening to staff.

A previously cooperative patient begins to refuse medications, is reluctant to eat and demands to go home.

Staff, especially nighttime staff, is accused of verbal and/or physical abuse. Often this takes the form of "they are trying to poison me."

A previously calm patient becomes agitated, is found wandering, or has frequent outbursts of crying.

When the delirious patient is seen by the psychiatrist the mental status examination typically reveals:

Decreased cognition, often with disorientation to time, and impaired recent memory.

Reduced capacity to focus and shift attention.

Decreased concentration.

Labile affect.

Paranoid thinking, sometimes with gross delusions or hallucinations.

In less medically ill patients who suffer from delirium, the underlying cause can usually be found, corrected and the delirium reversed. Typically in advanced cancer patients the single cause cannot be discovered and the delirium cannot be completely cured. However, usually the most distressing symptoms once treated can be relieved or greatly reduced. Low dose haloperidol (0.5mg - 2mg/day) is well tolerated and is very useful in the management of delirium in advanced cancer patients. It is especially useful if psychotic symptoms are present. A minor tranquilizer with a short half-life such as lorazepam can also be useful in treating the agitation that often is present in delirium. Consistent, reassuring interactions by visitors and staff, frequent orientation and familiar objects in the patients' room can also greatly reduce stress and discomfort. A clock and calendar can be useful and excessive stimulation should be avoided.

Health care professionals all too often believe that depression is a natural consequence of having a diagnosis of advanced cancer. This false assumption is usually rooted in a lack of understanding of depression as an illness and/or a manifestation of the caregiver's own sense of helplessness in caring for someone with advanced cancer. Consequently, there is a serious under treatment of depression which condemns a significant group of patients to suffer horrible psychic pain unnecessarily during the last phase of life.

Although advanced cancer patients commonly feel sad or depressed, in our experience less than 20% become clinically depressed. Major depression is an illness that is all pervasive and all consuming. Nothing is enjoyed. The patient is typically withdrawn or anxious. There is usually a feeling of hopelessness or helplessness and often the patient will believe that his illness is in some way punishment that is deserved. The wish to die is common and the risk of suicide can be high. Fortunately clinical depression, even in advanced cancer, can be effectively treated. The patient must be reassured that his depression is an illness that can and will improve. Frequent supportive encouragement by staff including nursing, social work, the attending physician, pastoral care and other team members is essential. The patient must be shown that he is valued and will not be abandoned.

Pharmacological intervention in major depression is almost always indicated. At Calvary Hospital the first line of antidepressant medications have become the SSRI's including fluoxetine (Prozac®), paroxetine (Paxil®) and sertraline (Zoloft®.) Tricylic antidepressants (TCA) are also effective in treating depression. When TCA is used, we suggest nortriptyline or desipramine because of fewer side effects than other TCAs. Our experience is that advanced cancer patients often respond more quickly and at relatively lower doses than physically healthy patients with depression. The undertreatment of depression in the advanced cancer patient is perhaps the single most serious shortcoming that continues to persist in this field.

Reference

1. Massie MJ, Holland J, Glass E. Delirium in terminally ill cancer patients. Am J Psychiatry 1983;140(8):pp 1040-58.

INTERCURRENT DISEASES
James E. Cimino

This topic refers to a combination of diseases occurring at the same time. Each may result in a fatal outcome or may be a nonfatal illness occurring in a patient who is already suffering from a fatal illness. The combinations are endless. First we need to reflect on the value of categorizing a patient as being near the end of life and whether or not it puts the patient in jeopardy of being denied an opportunity to benefit from treatment of the intercurrent illness.

As an example, I often relate the story about one of my first experiences at Calvary Hospital more than thirty-six years ago. A patient was referred for terminal care because of advanced cancer and presumed metastatic brain tumor. A routine urine analysis performed at the time of admission found the patient to be suffering from diabetic ketoacidosis in addition to the underlying "terminal" illness. The patient was treated for the diabetic acidosis and improved so dramatically that she was able to be discharged and survived comfortably for many months. She had been labeled "terminal" and while awaiting transfer the patient was only casually visited and inadequately examined on rounds in a teaching hospital. As a result, the progressive lethargy she experienced was attributed to the brain tumor. Although there are many examples in the literature[1,2,3] and over the years similar experiences at Calvary Hospital, it was that patient who has made me hesitant to label any patient "terminal" with the implication that nothing more could be done. I recognized that even in the so-called "terminal" patient there was always something that could be done. It was evident that applying the term "terminal" places the patient at risk of being abandoned. Thus, the articulation of the nonabandonment philosophy that we espouse at Calvary Hospital. The qualities embodied in the definition of nonabandonment are communication, removing the aura of fear, showing genuine concern, being available and above all, keeping promises. It also means being alert to the patient's physiological and psychological status in order to change the plan of treatment when indicated.

Among the more frequent and commonly treatable intercurrent illnesses that occur in patients near the end of life are diabetes mellitus, atrial fibrillation, congestive heart failure, renal failure and of course, a multitude of infections particularly of the urinary tract and lung. There are a myriad of other illnesses but these few examples demonstrate the dilemmas and principles in caring for these patients. I will avoid detailed discussion of the specific treatment of these diseases, but will outline general principles of care. Ideally, it is extremely important to obtain reasonable outcome statistics for any intervention when that is possible.

In the management of diabetes mellitus, euglycemia is rarely the goal of therapy for the near end of life patient.[4] Prevention of long term complications is no longer the goal. Diet can be liberalized and by accepting higher blood sugar levels both medication and frequent laboratory studies can be reduced. An additional benefit is the likelihood of avoiding the complication of hypoglycemia. This does not mean that one should not strive for some moderation in control of blood sugar. Blood sugars over 200mg per dl. can lead to a high incidence of infection and excessive hyperglycemia can cause an osmotic diuresis with its accompanying complications of dehydration and electrolyte abnormalities. Because the patient and family may have been counseled for years regarding the importance of rigid control of blood sugar, it is very important that the more liberal blood sugar control be explained to both the patient and the family.

The management of atrial fibrillation includes the use of anticoagulation. The overall statistical incidence of embolic phenomena secondary to untreated atrial fibrillation with anticoagulants is from 4.5 - 12% per patient-year.[5] However, the risk of thromboembolism by not anticoagulating these near end of life patients is of less concern when one realizes that they are unlikely to survive for even one year. It also removes the burden of following coagulation studies and the inherent risk of hemorrhage from the anticoagulant regimen.

Physicians are poor at predicting survival in patients with congestive heart failure.[6] On the other hand, heart failure causes significant symptoms and the management of congestive heart failure with ACE inhibitors, diuretics, possibly digoxin, vasodilators and even oxygen can usually be managed with minimal inconvenience to the patient. The patient's symptoms, heart rate, blood pressure and daily weights need to be measured and evaluated, but these measurements will not cause undo burden. Symptom relief is the goal and not necessarily prolongation of life. Therefore, if the chosen regimen should prove burdensome, it can be withdrawn.

Fundamental to the conservative management of renal failure is the use of a protein and potassium limited diet. These patients, in all likelihood, are already on a compromised diet that limits their protein. However, it may be necessary to restrict potassium so as not to cause an unnecessarily premature demise. This can usually be accomplished with little inconvenience to the patient. If the patient insists on consuming high potassium foods, it may be reasonable to add an oral exchange resin (Kayexalate) to the regimen. I would not recommend resin enemas for a debilitated near end of life patient. A review of the patient's medications is also in order, since some, such as ACE inhibitors and spironolactone can cause potassium retention.

Although antibiotics are readily available and usually easily administered, management of infection can still be burdensome for the patient and these burdens must be weighed carefully against the benefits that can be achieved. The cliché "pneumonia is an old man's (or woman's) best friend," does not always apply. One needs to know when the infection is part of the expected terminal event or when treatment can return the patient to his or her desired quality of life.

Each situation is unique. Treatment decisions must be weighed against the goal of the patient. What is the goal? Is it to stay alive as long as possible? Or is it to be comfortable even if it means a shortening of life? When treatment is refused, is it intended to cause death sooner or is it to avoid an undo burden of the treatment itself? This then becomes an ethical and even an emotional issue and must be answered within that context.

These are difficult choices. Accurate outcome data can make them easier. Good science should help craft informed decisions for these patients by uncovering accurate data and clearly explaining the risks and burdens of treatments.

References

1. Bell B. Pseudo-terminal patients make comeback. Medical World News, August 12, 1966; pp 108-109.

2. Taube W, Jenkins C, Bruera E. Is a "palliative" patient always a palliative patient? Two case studies. J Pain Symptom Manag 1997;13: pp 347-351.

3. Potter JF. A challenge for the hospice movement. N Eng J Med 1980;302: pp 53-55.

4. Poulson J. The management of diabetes in patients with advanced cancer. J Pain Sympt Manag 1997;13: pp 339-346.

5. Kearon C, Hirsh J. Management of anticoagulation before and after elective surgery. N Eng J Med 1997; 336: pp 1506-1511.

6. Poses RM, Smith WR, McClish DK, et al. Physicians' survival predictions for patients with acute congestive heart failure. Arch Int Med 1997;157: pp 1001-07.

CHEMOTHERAPY: ITS PLACE IN PALLIATIVE CARE – BREAST, PROSTATE, PANCREAS, MULTIPLE MYELOMA
David I. Wollner

Systemic chemotherapy can play a vital role in treatment of advanced neoplastic disease. Cure can be attained in most patients with gestational trophoblastic disease (GTN), non-seminomatous germ cell tumors (NSGCT), and Hodgkin's. More commonly, objective responses using a combination of agents translate into extension of survival and improvement in quality of life (QOL). Often a partial response may not improve survival but may enhance QOL; metastatic large bowel cancer is a prime example. Most incurable neoplasms such as malignant melanoma, renal cell carcinoma, hepatocellular carcinoma, and others show no objective response to systemic chemo-therapy.

An objective response is the standard tool in new drug studies. More recently a large number of QOL tools have been added to definitions of clinical efficacy regardless of objective response. Examples are the Memorial Pain Assessment Card (MPAC), and the European Organization for Research and Treatment of Cancer (EORTC) Quality of Life Questionnaire (QOLQ.) The latter is ideal for studies in a palliative care setting.

Candidate Selection

The following criteria favorably select candidates for systemic chemotherapy:

A good performance status: KPS >50 (Karnofsky Performance Status)
ECOG <3 (Eastern Cooperative Oncology Group)
Adequate organ function:
    Bone marrow; HGB > 9.0 gm %; WBC > 3.0×10^3
    Plts > 100×10^3; Kidney
    BUN < 2x NL (Blood Urea Nitrogen)
    Cr. ≤ 1.5 mgm/dl (Creatinine)
    Liver; Transaminases < 2x NL
    Bilirubin < 2x NL; Albumin > 3.5 gm/dl
Clinically controlled co-morbidities (e.g., CHF, infection)
No prior chemotherapy
Informed consent

Assessment of Efficacy

Response to systemic chemotherapy is assessed objectively and/or subjectively. Objective responses occur with bi-dimensionally measurable disease (e.g., pulmonary metastases) or with evaluable disease (e.g., hepatomegaly.) The ideal goal is to attain a complete remission (CR), (fig. 1) as any other level would not lead to a cure.

DEFINITION OF RESPONSES AFTER CHEMOTHERAPY[1]

Complete remission: Disappearance of all signs and symptoms, or recalcification of all osteolytic metastases for at least one month

Partial remission: Decrease, by more than 50%, of the sum of the products of the two largest perpendicular diameters of all measurable lesions, in the absence of growth of any lesion or appearance of a new lesion

Stable disease: no significant change in tumor size or any signs or symptoms caused by the tumor

Progression: increase of more than 25% in lesion size or appearance of new lesions

Breast

Hormonal therapy, additive or ablative, is the first choice for systemic therapy for metastatic disease. From 1 to 2/3rds of patients show an objective response and toxicities are minimal. Systemic chemotherapy is reserved for disease refractory to hormones or initially aggressive receptor-negative disease with visceral metastases. The number of effective agents and their combinations is vast. The anthracyclines and/or taxanes should form the base of a given regimen.

If a patient is eligible, one of two protocols can be used:

Doxorubicin 10mg/m^2 slow IV push once weekly

Weekly assessment should reveal a response in <6 weeks. The total dose should not to exceed 450 mg/m^2. Cardiomyopathy is a rare, irreversible event (seen in less than 5% of patients).

Taxanes. Paclitaxel 175 mg/m^2 IV over 3 hours or Docetaxel 100 mg/m^2 IV over 3 hours

Premedication with a corticosteroid and an H-2 blocker is required. Blood pressure must be monitored each 15 minutes during infusion. Rapidly developing neutropenia may occur and G-CSF (Granulocyte Colony Stimulating Factor) should be available. A response is usually seen within 4 weeks

Prostate

The standard therapy of symptomatic, advanced local disease is bilateral surgical orchiectomy or the use of a GnRH agonist and an antiandrogen. The primary principle of therapy is androgen deprivation although total androgen blockade (TAB) has not been proven to be superior to the two modalities cited.

Hormone refractory disease eventually develops. A hormone withdrawal response should be assessed as second-line hormonal therapy is not commonly effective.

There are a few agents that reveal marginal activity in hormonally refractory tumors. However one protocol can be used -- Mitoxantrone 12 mg/m^2 IVP every three weeks and prednisone 5.0mg PO BID daily chronically. Mitoxantrone has cumulative cardiotoxicity. Appreciation of acute and chronic toxicities of prednisone is required, including delirium, hyperglycemia, myopathy.

Pancreas

There is no effective standard therapy for this disease; it is rarely curable. Five-fluorouracil is considered "standard" therapy but after 40 years of study and the wide variability of responses with no survival advantage, this term is inaccurate.

Although advanced disease is measurable, at times subjective symptoms are very common: pain, weight loss, and fatigue. Gemcitabine is a bis-fluorinated antipyrimidine that inhibits DNA and RNA synthesis. In open and randomized studies this agent provided a statistically significant clinical benefit response (when evaluating pain, opioid consumption, KPS and weight gain.) Additionally when compared to 5-FU, a survival advantage is seen. In patients with regionally advanced disease and/or distant metastases with a life expectancy of >12 weeks and no prior chemotherapy, a protocol could be considered consisting of Gemcitabine 1.0 gm/m^2, slow IV infusion, weekly. QOL tools must be applied weekly and CBC and serum transaminases must be monitored monthly. Efficacy can be determined within 8 weeks.

Multiple Myeloma

Multiple myeloma is a plasma cell neoplasm in which systemic chemotherapy improves survival and enhances QOL. Bone pain, hypercalcemia and spinal cord compression are common symptoms of Stage III disease. Although high dose chemotherapy with bone marrow support may produce prolonged remissions, standard chemotherapy is the proven means used to achieve clinical success.

L-phenylanine mustard (LPAM) and prednisone can be tried in previously untreated patients. LPAM 8mg/m^2 is administered orally every 4 weeks and prednisone 2 mg/m^2 orally daily for 5 consecutive days every 4 weeks, given HS on an empty stomach Delayed myelosuppression is seen requiring biweekly monitoring of neutrophil and platelet counts. Objective and subjective parameters must be followed monthly. Pain and opioid equivalent consumption includes: "M" protein titer, Serial HGB, BUN/CR, and calcium. Appreciation of acute and chronic toxicities of prednisone is required (as in carcinoma of the prostate.)

Conclusion

As the spectrum of patients with incurable neoplastic disease widens, systemic chemotherapy will be rarely used. With precise assessment and selection, patients with incurable carcinomas and multiple myelomas may have enhanced an improved QOL.

CHEMOTHERAPY: ITS PLACE IN PALLIATIVE CARE – LUNG, COLORECTAL, NON-HODGKIN'S LYMPHOMAS
Devmani Jaitly

Lung Cancer

Lung cancer represents a major health epidemic worldwide and is one of the most common causes of cancer death both in males and females. Most patients present with disseminated disease and only a few can be cured. Patients with incurable lung cancer require comfort and palliation. Various options are available. Management plans apply equally both to small and non-small cell cancer since morbidity is considered to be similar in all forms of the disease.

Disseminated disease can include bone, brain, liver, and the lung itself. Patients often have severe dyspnea, hemoptysis and other symptoms relating to pulmonary insufficiency. Obstructive symptomatology as well as infections occur. These distressors can often be relieved with opioids, antibiotics, corticosteroids, and palliative radiation. A majority of patients with bone metastases obtain pain relief with radiation in conjunction with opioid therapy. Radiation complications are not a deterrent factor because of the short life expectancy. Much of the decision-making in the treatment of such patients depends upon his/her performance status. For example, patients with good status can be offered surgical orthopedic procedures if lytic lesions are noted in the weight-bearing bones.

Chemotherapy plays a minor role since no significant prolongation of life nor symptom improvement have been noted. Patients with poor status are at far greater risk of lethal toxicity even when treated with modest chemotherapy doses. Agents considered include cytoxan, cisplatinum, paclitaxel and etoposide. Newer agents include carboplatin, vinorelbine, docetaxel, gemcitabine, and irinotecan. Carboplatin causes less nausea and vomiting than cisplatinum and is easier to administer.

A thorough discussion should be carried out with the patient and family prior to administration of these agents. Emphasis should be placed on the toxicity profiles and the fact that no significant life prolongation may be achieved. The toxicity of cytoxan includes bone marrow depression and hemorrhagic cystitis. Cisplatin causes renal damage, nausea, vomiting, electrolyte disturbances, peripheral neuropathy, and bone marrow depression. Carboplatin causes bone marrow depression, nausea, vomiting, and peripheral neuropathy. Paclitaxil causes bone marrow depression, nausea, vomiting, and alopecia. Etoposide causes bone marrow depression, nausea, vomiting, diarrhea, and hypotension. Most of these agents cause bone marrow depression and the resulting complications can be very difficult to treat. Any "aggressive" treatment should be undertaken with extreme caution.

Treatment modalities to be considered include palliation for pain, dyspnea, infectious complications, obstruction, hemoptysis, bleeding, and cough. Chemotherapy can be overwhelming. Family support is extremely important at this time in the patient's life.

Colorectal Cancer

Each year approximately 155,000 new cases of colorectal cancer are diagnosed in the United States. Colorectal cancer is the third most common malignancy after lung and prostate cancer in men and after lung and breast cancer in women. The overall incidence of this malignancy is nearly identical in both sexes. These statistics are reflected in our patient population. Familial colorectal cancer syndromes include heredity polyposis and non-polyposis cancer. Other high risk illnesses include inflammatory bowel diseases, ulcerative colitis and Crohn's disease. The majority of patients have no clear predisposing conditions.

The most commonly used staging system for colorectal cancer is the Duke's staging system:

Stage A: tumor penetration confined to the mucosa of the intestine
Stage B1: tumor penetration into the muscular layer
Stage B2: tumor penetration through muscle into the serosa or the perirectal fat;
Stage C1 & C2: Duke's Stages B1 & B2, with lymph node involvement
Stage D: distant metastatic disease.

The pattern of metastatic spread is different for rectal and colon cancer. Colon cancer typically metastasizes to the regional nodes and liver via the portal system. Patients often present in advanced stages with liver failure and symptoms of metabolic encephalopathy or clinical problems secondary to multiorgan failure.

Patients with lower rectal cancer tend to develop lung metastases because the venous drainage of the distal rectum is through the inferior and medial hemorrhoidal veins which are not part of the portal circulation. Rectal carcinoma patients may have changes in bowel habits, rectal fullness, urgency and bleeding. Pelvic pain usually indicates local extension of the tumor. Some patients present with abdominal obstruction including nausea and vomiting.

Therapy

Surgery is the primary treatment for these tumors. For colon carcinoma hemicolectomy is the treatment of choice. For rectal carcinomas, low inferior or abdominal perineal resections may be indicated depending upon the tumor's location. In our patients, chemotherapy is rarely indicated because of the disease's advanced nature of the disease and poor patient performance status. The most effective single agent in the management of advanced colorectal cancer is 5-fluorouracil but it is rarely indicated alone. Adjuvant therapy for Duke's Stage C colon cancer includes therapy with 5 fluorouracil and levamisole. Surgery may play a role for solitary or several liver metastases confined to one lobe of the liver. For other metastatic disease standard chemotherapy combines 5-fluorouracil and levamisole. Several other regimens are available but they have little overall effect on survival. Adjuvant treatment for rectal cancer should include a combination of radiation therapy with chemotherapy.

Patients with advanced tumors suffer from sumptoms of multiorgan failure such as anemia, weakness, anorexia, fatigue, abdominal pain and discomfort. Chapters on gastrointestinal obstruction, nausea, vomiting, pain and blood transfusion discuss specific management of the symptoms that arise. In all our patients, control of these symptoms is paramount. [1,2]

Non-Hodgkin's Lymphomas

The Non-Hodgkin's lymphomas constitute a heterogenous group of lympho proliferative disorders usually associated with varied survival and a prognosis related to the histopathology. Lymphomas can be broadly understood as being of three grades: low, intermediate, and high grade malignancy. The working formulation of the Non-Hodgkin's lymphomas is contained in the list below.

Working Formulation	% In Adults
Low Grade:	
Diffuse, small lymphocytic	4
Follicular, mixed small cleaved and large cell	8
Follicular, predominantly small cleaved cell	23
Intermediate Grade:	
Follicular, predominantly large cell	4
Diffuse, small cleaved cell	7
Diffuse, mixed small and large cell	7
Diffuse, large cell	20
High Grade:	
Large cell immunoblastic	8
Lymphoblastic	4
Small noncleaved	5
Miscellaneous	10

The most common B cell neoplasms in the Western hemisphere are follicular lymphomas but less common in other areas of the world. They comprise approximately 45% of the non-Hodgkins lymphomas and about 80% of all indolent lymphomas. These follicular lymphomas have a median survival of 8-10 years.[3]

Ann Arbor Staging System For Non-Hodgkin's Lymphomas

Stage I - A single lymph-node region or extra lymphatic site.

Stage II - Two or more lymph-node regions on the same side of the diaphragm or localized extra lymphatic site with one or more lymph-node regions on the same side of the diaphragm.

Stage III - Lymph-node regions on both sides of the diaphragm and possible localized involvement of an extralymphatic site or the spleen.

Stage IV - Disseminated involvement of one or more extralymphatic organs or tissues.

A or B denotes absence (A) or presence (B) of unexplained weight loss > 10%, unexplained fever > 38°C, or night sweats. (Note: pruritus is not a B symptom)

Some of the clinical findings noted in lymphomas are related to lymph node enlargement, especially bulky masses in the neck or the retro-peritoneum. Spleno-megaly is not common in the follicular lymphomas. Mediastinal lymph node involvement may occur but superior vena caval syndrome is unlikely. Other findings may include anemia and sometimes leukemic transformation. Abdominal pain and discomfort may be noted secondary to lymph node involvement and change in bowel habits or GI bleeding. Imaging studies of chest, abdomen and pelvis are indicated to assess the degree of lymph node involvement. Lymphangiography is used less often because of the availability of other more sensitive imaging modalities.

Prognostic factors are important in assessing lymphomas. Laboratory criteria indicating a poor prognosis include elevation of the serum LDH, an increased expression of the nuclear proliferation antigen KI 67 and an increased percentage of cells in the S phase. The clinical course of these lymphomas varies; some patients experience a very aggressive disease while others may have a prolonged and indolent course. The majority of patients with advanced low grade non-Hodgkins lymphoma respond to initial chemotherapy. Virtually all patients ultimately relapse and most die of their disease.

A number of factors may influence the treatment decision for a patient with a newly diagnosed indolent lymphoma including the histology and his/her performance status. Sometimes a watch-and-wait policy is considered acceptable in asymptomatic patients. Older patients, with poor performance status and those with other serious medical problems can be considered for oral chemotherapeutic agents. In the advanced stages, a patient must be monitored for symptoms including pain, seizures, dehydration and declining performance status. They are prone to multiple infections. Chemotherapeutic agents are usually not indicated. In advanced stages, a leukemic transformation may occur. This is considered a worsening of the histopathology of lymphoma toward an aggressive type.

Richter transformation is the development of diffuse large cell lymphoma in patients with a history of chronic lymphocytic leukemia or other low grade well differentiated lymphomas. This is more aggressive than the usual large cell lymphoma and has an extremely poor prognosis.

The intermediate and high grade non-Hodgkins lymphomas also carry a poor prognosis. The clinical manifestations are diverse and depend on the site of the disease. These tumors grow rapidly and present as masses that cause symptoms when the infiltrate tissues or obstruct organs and are more frequently localized. Sites of involvement include the lymph nodes, spleen, liver, bone marrow, and skin. The GI tract may be involved and manifests in the mucosa lymphoid tissue. Pain within an enlarged lymph node is also seen in a rapidly growing tumor.

The systemic features include presentation of the B symptoms including fever, drenching night sweats, and more than 10% weight loss. Generalized pruritus may also be present. Paraneoplastic syndromes may occur. Hypercalcemia is seen in about 10% of the patients. Prognostic factors include age, B symptoms, the performance status of the patient, the extent of the tumor burden, the Ann Arbor stage number of extra nodal sites, serum LDH level and the serum B_2 micro globulin level.

In view of the high grade histopathology and aggressive nature of the illness, these patients are treated with a combination chemotherapy regimen. Unfortunately relapse is common. Radiation therapy is also used and recently bone marrow transplantation protocols have been explored and recommended accordingly.[4]

Conclusion

Chemotherapeutic intervention in the advanced disease stage is largely nonproductive. No realistic life prolongation can be expected. Patients should be monitored for development of the leukemic phase or cytopenia. Infections can be treated and transfusions can be provided when carefully considering the goal intended. These patients have undergone tremendous stress and need sympathetic and made comfortable requiring meticulous nursing care.

References

1. Beahrs OH, Myers MH, eds. American Joint Committee on Cancer. Manual for staging of cancer. 3rd ed. Philadelphia: JB Lippincott, 1983.

2. DeVita VT, Hellman S, Rosenberg SA (eds). Cancer: principles and practice of oncology. 4th ed. Philadelphia, PA: JB Lippincott, 1993.

3. Berard CW, Bloomfield C, Bonadonna G, et al. Classifications of non-Hodgkins lymphomas reproducibility of major classification systems. Cancer 1985;55:91-95.

4. Rosenberg SA. Karnofsky Memorial Lecture. The low-grade non-Hodgkin's lymphomas:challenges and opportunities. J Clin Oncol 1985;3:299.

RADIOTHERAPY
Flora Mincer

External beam radiation treatment is a well established, simple and effective means of relieving many diverse local symptoms of primary or metastatic cancer. Side effects of radiation are minimal as used in this palliative care setting. Treatment indications can be categorized as follows:

The high frequency of bone metastases which occur in a wide variety of malignancies make bone pain the most frequent indication for palliative radiotherapy. In addition to relief of pain, early intervention may prevent fracture

Pain resulting from spinal or peripheral nerve compression by osseous, lymphatic or visceral cancer growth will respond to radiation in as high as 80% of cases

The major radiotherapy emergency is spinal cord compression. This is most frequently seen in the dorsal spine; intervention within 6 - 12 hours markedly increases probability of complete functional recovery

Vascular obstruction by primary or metastatic carcinoma may be ameliorated or reversed, e.g., in superior vena caval syndrome, or peripheral lymphatic obstruction due to inguinal/iliac or axillary adenopathy

Visceral obstruction (e.g. esophageal, bronchial, ureteral) may be effectively relieved by radiation

Hemorrhage, especially from small vessels, is a frequent indication for palliative radiation for lung, uterine, rectal or bladder carcinomas. Bleeding, ulcerating skin cancers and primary breast cancers may regress and ultimately may even re-epithelialize after radiotherapy.

Several examples are described below showing the desirable and sometimes dramatic treatment results that are possible with the limited facilities and treatment schedules used at Calvary Hospital.

1) SYP was a 68 year old woman with lung carcinoma and a huge destructive femoral metastasis with extension into surrounding soft tissue of the thigh. Radiation treatment: 2 doses of 8 Gy resulted in 75% reduction in the externally visible and palpable mass and marked pain reduction for the entire duration of her last six weeks of life.

2) EE was an 82 year old woman with generalized large cell lymphoma and cranial nerve involvement. She received 25 Gy in 7 fractions to the base of the

skull including cranial nerves with complete resolution of cranial nerve palsies and complete clearing of lesions on repeat MRI.

3) JG was a middle-aged man with a rapidly expanding carcinoma of the lung causing hemorrhage which required blood transfusions. Radiation treatment to a total dose of 24 Gy in 6 fractions resulted in complete arrest of bleeding and significant reduction in lung mass enabling the patient to return to his home.

4) FM was a 30 year old man with recurrent aggressive disseminated Hodgkin's disease and excruciating bone pain. Several bone areas were treated with marked pain relief enabling him to leave Calvary Hospital for many months.

The Radiotherapy Department at Calvary Hospital was established in the mid-1960s with the installation of a Cobalt Teletherapy Unit. The present Cobalt machine, designed to treat at 60 - 80 cm., is used almost exclusively at the standard 80 cm. SSD. The machine head can be angled in all directions and accommodates a stretcher or bed, thus minimizing painful patient transfers.

The dose regimen established to maximize prompt benefit in patients with a life expectancy under six months has been a so-called hypo-fractionation schedule. Single or a few relatively high radiation doses are applied once or twice per week usually for one to three treatments. Most patients receive a dose of 6-8 Gy (i.e., 600-800 cGy or rad) measured at the skin ("given dose" or d_{max}). More recently the doses have been calculated at the depth. These range from 4 to 8 Gy depending on tumor and field size, depth of tumor and risk to vulnerable underlying organs. Comparative studies with standard fractionation (30 - 40 Gy in 2 - 4 weeks) have shown comparable acute benefit without undue side effects in a number of palliative situations. We have not had any notable complications from the hypo-fractionation regimen.

We do not have facilities for either the administration of Sr89 radio-isotope or for "hemi-body" large field radiation, both of which are useful in certain patients with widespread bone metastases. Those patients who might benefit from such treatments are referred to a regional acute care facility.

Comprehensive surveys of palliative radiotherapy are listed in the references.

References

1. Hoskin PJ. Radiotherapy in symptom management. In: Doyle D, et al. Textbook of Palliative Care. New York: Oxford University Press 1994; pp 117-22.

2. Hogle D. Current problems in cancer. 1997; Vol. 21: pp 129-84.

HYPERCALCEMIA
Michael Eufemio

Hypercalcemia is a common occurrence in the advanced cancer patient -- particularly in those with multiple myeloma, lung and breast malignancies. These patients require certain modifications of the drugs used, dosage and routes of administration.

Acute Hypercalcemia

Acute hypercalcemia has been variably defined by an absolute total serum calcium, greater than 13 mg/dl, when corrected for the serum albumin. Ionized calcium, however, is considered to be preferable to the total serum calcium since it is the physiologically critical value and is not affected by abnormalities in serum proteins (hypoalbuminemia or hypergammaglobulinemia as in myeloma, or abnormalities in acid base status with altered calcium binding to protein, i.e., acidosis decreases binding of ionized calcium to protein.) However, we have found that the admittedly crude correction of calcium for the albumin level (0.8 mg/dl for deviation of 1.0 grams/dl albumin from normal) to be adequate in the diagnosis of hypercalcemia and establishing criteria for therapy.

Patients can be asymptomatic with calciums above 13 mg/dl but some can be symptomatic with calcium levels much less than 13 mg/dl. Many of the Calvary patients fall into this latter category and therefore, therapy for acute hypercalcemia must be determined not only by the absolute value of the serum calcium, but also by the clinical condition of the patient.

Therapeutic Recommendations

Intravenous hydration represents the universally accepted initial therapy for hypercalcemia and is mandatory since almost all patients who are acutely hypercalcemic are dehydrated.[1,2] Dehydration results in decreased renal calcium clearance and worsening of the hypercalcemia. Although intravenous hydration does not correct the basic underlying mechanism of hypercalcemia, i.e., bone resorption, and cannot be used indefinitely, it permits stabilization of the patient until other therapeutic modalities can be introduced. Almost any fluid will be effective in correcting the dehydration. The amount of IV fluids must be adjusted according to the renal and cardiopulmonary status of the patient. We use dextrose in water rather than saline in our patients who have severely compromised cardiorenal function. Despite the lack of the osmotic sodium diuresis and the competitive sodium inhibition of calcium reabsorption provided by saline solutions, we have found that dextrose in water is almost as effective as a means of hydration as saline.

Drug Therapy

Diuretics:

Loop diuretics, such as Lasix, are usually used with IV saline to promote a sodium and water diuresis and decrease the sodium load that may cause congestive heart failure. However, it should not be given unless the patient is adequately hydrated, i.e., has received at least two to three liters of fluids. If given without adequate hydration, it will worsen the dehydration and the hypercalcemia. Serum potassium must be monitored closely with the loop diuretics, and if the patient is on digitalis the dose should be lowered or temporarily discontinued, particularly if hypokalemia occurs.

Mithramycin (plicamycin):

This antineoplastic drug was once considered to be the drug of choice for the treatment of hypercalcemia. Its mechanism of action is inhibition of the synthesis of messenger RNA (not tumor destruction) resulting ultimately in decreased osteoclastic activity. However, compared to the newer drug therapies, it is a relatively more toxic drug with the potential for bone marrow suppression, hepatic and renal toxicity and bleeding even with a normal platelet count. We use this drug only for refractory hypercalcemia.

Calcitonin:

The anti-osteoclastic action of calcitonin has been utilized for years in the treatment of hypercalcemia and is a particularly good drug for our patients.[3,4] There are no significant hepatic, renal or hematological toxicities and only mild side effects of nausea, vomiting, flushing and headache. In a dose of up to 8 MRC units/kg q 6 hours, giving a patient 200-400 units IM or IV q 4- 6 hours, serum calcium will decrease in 12 to 24 hours. It will also cause increased renal excretion of calcium immediately after administration, an effect not shared by the other anti-osteoclastic agents to be discussed. Therefore, even if continuous therapy with calcitonin is not used, we recommend its initial use for its calciuretic effect. Unfortunately patients often become refractory to its calcium-lowering effect due to either development of anti-calcitonin antibodies or down regulation of calcitonin receptors. This effect may be prevented or delayed by the concomitant use of glucocorticoids along with the calcitonin.

Glucocorticoid:

Glucocorticoids are effective therapy for hypercalcemia for certain tumors.[5] They decrease gastrointestinal absorption of calcium (possibly due to antagonism of Vitamin D), increase glomerular filtration rate, increase renal excretion of calcium, acutely decrease efflux of calcium from bone (possibly by antagonism of the action of PTH on bone) and by direct anti-tumor effects. However, the availability of diphosphonates has made this therapy almost obsolete. They may still be employed as adjunctive therapy in cases of refractory hypercalcemia, particularly in patients with multiple myeloma and breast cancer with bone metastases. Steroids are most effective in patients with bone lesions rather than in patients with humoral hypercalcemia of malignancy. They are also very effective in patients with Hodgkins' disease, lymphoma and malignancies associated with production of 1- 25 dihydroxy Vitamin D and osteoclast activating factors (lymphokines.)

Disphosphonates:

Disphosphonates are analogs of pyrophosphate whose anti-resorptive action is attributed to inhibition of osteoclastic activity and also by making the hydroxyapatite crystal of bone more resistant to dissolution.[4,6,7] They are now considered to be the calcium-lowering drugs of choice with no serious toxicity and only minimal side effects. A flu-like syndrome with low-grade fever may occur for one to two days after therapy. The newer diphosphonate - Aredia (pamidronate) is an ideal drug for our patients. It can be given in the recommended total dose of 60-90 mg with one infusion over 12-24 hours. Initially, the dose varied from 30-90 mg depending on the degree of hypercalcemia, but we use the full 90 mg dose, since like all diphosphonates, it is relatively free of serious side effects. The onset of the antihypercalcemic response occurs in 24 to 48 hours and normocalcemia can be maintained for an average of one to three weeks before another dose is required.

Diphosphonates can be used in full doses even in patients with chronic renal insufficiency since recent studies have shown no adverse side effects, even in anuric dialysis patients with hypercalcemia.[8,9]

Inorganic Phosphorous:

Inorganic phosphorous is no longer considered appropriate for the treatment of acute hypercalcemia since there is no IV preparation available. However in certain settings, oral phosphorous such as Fleet's Phosphosoda or Nutraphos (1 g of elemental phosphorous/4-5 g phosphate salt) in doses of 2-3 grams of elemental phosphorous a day can be used in a patient able to swallow medications. There is less danger of metastatic calcification occurring with oral inorganic phosphorous.

Since patients with chronic renal disease may develop marked hyperphosphatemia with a calcium-phosphorous product exceeding 80 (and resulting metastatic calcifications) it is best used in patients with a normal BUN and creatinine and low serum phosphorous level (less than 3.0.) These criteria often exclude many of our patients.

Gallium nitrate:

Gallium nitrate, another antiresorptive agent, is effective in the therapy of hypercalcemia, but its renal toxicity has made it a less desirable choice.[7]

Combination therapy is often needed to decrease serum calcium particularly when they exert a synergistic effect.

Therapy of Chronic and Recurrent Hypercalcemia

Whereas the therapy of acute hypercalcemia is usually very successful, the maintenance of normocalcemia and the therapy of chronic, mild hypercalcemia has been disappointing. The lack of serious side effects of parenteral diphosphonates, on the other hand, would make the use of oral diphosphonates theoretically an ideal form of therapy to maintain a normal serum calcium. We have embarked upon a study of the use of Fosamax (alendronate) in the prevention of recurrent hypercalcemic events following normalization of serum calcium with IV Aredia. If this proves to be more effective than oral Didronel or Clodronate, it will reduce the need for repeated infusions of Aredia enabling patients to remain out of the hospital for longer periods of time.

The Decision to Treat Hypercalcemia in Malignant Disease

As with all aspects of the treatment of patients with advanced malignancies, certain philosophical issues are invariably raised when considering treatment of medical conditions due to or associated with advanced malignancies. The symptoms of hypercalcemia such as anorexia, nausea, vomiting, constipation, and abnormalities in cognitive function can be alleviated. Therefore, the decision to treat hypercalcemia should be based not on whether therapy will affect life expectancy, but rather on the need to relieve symptoms of hypercalcemia and to improve quality of life.

References

1. Ralston SL. Medical management of hypercalcemia. Br J Clin Pharmacol 1992; 34: pp 11-20.

2. Bilezikian JP. Management of hypercalcemia. J Clin Endo Metab 1993; 77: pp 1445-49.

3. Wisneski LA. Salmon calcitonin in the acute management of hypercalcemia. Calcified Tissue Intl 1990; 46 (Suppl):S26-530.

4. Fatami S, Singer RF, Rude RK. Effect of salmon calcitonin and etidronate on hypercalcemia of malignancy. Calc Tissue Intl 1992; 50: pp 107-09.

5. Kristensen B, Holmegaard SN, Transbol I, Mouridsen H. Prednisolone in the treatment of severe hypercalcemia in metastatic breast cancer. A randomized study. J Intern Med 1992; 232: pp 237-45.

6. Wimalawansa SJ. Optimal frequency of administration of pamidronte in patients with hypercalcemia of malignancy. Clin Endo 1994; 41: pp 591-95.

7. Warrell RP, Murphy WK, Schulman P, Odwyer PJ, Heller G. A randomized double-blind study of calcium nitrate compared with etidronate for acute control of cancer-related hypercalcemia. J Clin Oncol 1991; 9: pp 1467-75.

8. Davenport A. Treatment of hypercalcaemia with pamidronate in patients with end stage renal failure. Scandinavian J of Urol Neph 1993; 27:447-51.

9. Vap AS. Use of aminohydroxypropylidene biphosphonate (AHPrBP, "APD") for the treatment of hypercalcemia in patients with renal impairment. Clin Neph 1990; 34 (5):225-29.

AIDS
Dial Hewlett, Jr.

AIDS and malignancy have been linked since the initial descriptions of the new syndrome in 1981 when a cluster of young gay men in New York City were diagnosed with a previously rare malignancy known as Kaposi's Sarcoma.

Malignancies are a frequent cause of morbidity and mortality among individuals with AIDS.[1] Although the incidence of the most common AIDS associated neoplasm (Kaposi's Sarcoma) has dropped since the early part of the epidemics when it was found in nearly 47% of HIV infected patients, it currently is still diagnosed in 9% of patients with AIDS.[2] Non-Hodgkin's lymphoma (NHL), is the next most common AIDS associated malignancy and occurs in <1%. There is also an increased incidence of several other neoplastic diseases in individuals with HIV/AIDS. These include Hodgkin's Disease, cervical carcinoma, anorectal carcinoma, testicular carcinoma, small cell carcinoma, basal cell carcinoma, and melanoma. Co-infection with Human Papilloma (HPL) is strongly correlated with cervical and anorectal carcinomas.

Approximately 40% of patients with AIDS, will have disease courses complicated by the occurrence of a malignancy.[1] Antiretroviral therapy and antibiotic prophylactic regimens directed against pneumocystis pneumonia and disseminated mycobacterium avium complex infections (MAC) have resulted in remarkable improvements in the overall survival rates of patients with HIV.[3] Moreover, the quality of life is greatly enhanced by the utilization of combination Antiretroviral therapy. In many instances, the progression of malignant neoplasms particularly Kaposi's Sarcoma and certain lymphomas can be curtailed and in some instances reversed when regimens which include protease inhibitors are employed.

With the advent of the AIDS epidemic in the early 1980's and with New York City at the national epicenter of this devastating outbreak, patients with AIDS associated malignancies were encountered with increased frequency at Calvary Hospital. Traditionally, the major emphasis in the care of patients has been the provision of palliative and supportive care. Since the advent of protease inhibitors in late 1995 and the remarkable responses documented in many patients with even advanced stages of illness,[3] it became apparent that the development of a structured approach to these patients needed to be developed specifically addressing the following general areas: Clinical indications for Antiretroviral combination therapy. When should therapy be instituted or changed in patients transferred to our institution? How should patients on therapy be monitored while at Calvary? When is it appropriate to discontinue combination therapy? What types of regimens for antibiotic prophylaxis should be employed by the physicians at Calvary. Which patients are candidates for these regimens? How should these patients be monitored? When is it appropriate to discontinue therapy?

In 1987, we were encouraged by the results of the 019 trial in which patients with AIDS were placed into blinded trial and treated with either zidovudine (AZT) or placebo. The study was never completed because an interim analysis revealed excessive deaths among patients receiving placebo.[4] It was felt that continuation of the trial was unethical and subsequently, AZT was approved for general use in HIV infected patients with CD4 counts below 200. As time progressed, it became abundantly clear that long term, single drug antiretroviral therapy was ineffective and importantly might be contributing to the emergence of resistant strains of HIV. Emphasis in AIDS care abruptly shifted to antibiotic prophylaxis against common opportunistic infections particularly pneumocystitis which, in the late 1980's and early 1900's occurred in 65% of patients with advanced AIDS. Since routine use of trimethoprim/ sulfamethoazole prophylaxis therapy has become commonplace in the treatment of individuals with HIV, rates of pneumocystis have dropped significantly. Other forms of prophylaxis directed against fungal infections and mycobacterial infections have exerted a tremendous impact upon the morbidity and mortality among patients with AIDS.

Nearly all of the patients at Calvary are referred from surrounding area acute care hospitals. The incidence of malignancy complicating the course of AIDS may range from 5% to 40%. Earlier studies appear to have a much higher incidence largely due to Kaposi's sarcoma. Savona analyzed the experience with AIDS and malignancy in a hospital in the Bronx which serves as a referral source for Calvary.[5] They retrospectively reviewed 890 cases of AIDS presenting over a four year period between 1989 and 1993 and found that cancer was diagnosed and confirmed histologically in 46 patients (5%). Kaposi's sarcoma was the most common, occurring in eight patients. The median survival of these patients was twelve months.

At another New York City medical center, malignant neoplasia complicated AIDS in 12% of 869 cases occurring over an eight year period.[6] The gastrointestinal tract was involved in 32% of these patients with AIDS associated malignancy.

Plan for Treatment

At Calvary Hospital we recommend that each physician devise a therapeutic plan for each patient with an HIV/AIDS associated malignancy. This plan should be divided into three basic categories:

Palliative care (pain control/analgesia, comfort and nutritional support

Antimicrobial prophylaxis

Antiretroviral therapy.

General Palliative Care Issues

The medication list and schedules of patients with long-standing AIDS are often daunting and intimidating to the internist or family practitioner charged with the patient's care. In many cases, duplication exists and in some situations, drug interactions may actually be contributing to the patient's illness. In some cases inanition and dehydration are exacerbated by over zealous use of medication.

Severe painful neuritis may be caused by some of the nucleosides such as ddC (Hivid), d4T (Stavudine/Zerit®), and less frequently by AZT. Discontinuation of these agents may result in gradual relief of neuritis. Some success has been achieved with concurrent use of pyridoxine 50-100mg daily and in some cases amitriptyline (Elavil®). Quinine compounds may also be helpful.

Approximately 15% of patients receiving Epivir® (3TC) report severe headache. Combinations of fluconazole and rifabutin may cause visual disturbances while some of the antimicrobials particularly metronidazole and clarithromycin may be associated with taste perversion which can contribute to loss of appetite. The fluoroquinolone antibiotics lower seizure threshold and may make seizure disorders associated with CNS lesions more difficult to control. Persistent unexplained fever is sometimes caused by long term use of trimethoprim/sulfamethoxazole or dapsone.

A careful review of the medication list alongside a list of the patient's major complaints is time well spent.

Antimicrobial Prophylaxis

Antibiotic prophylaxis is a basic cornerstone of HIV/AIDS care and has contributed greatly to the increased rates of survival. In general, patients with CD4 counts >200 do not require prophylaxis for opportunistic infections such as pneumocystis. Patients with CD4 counts <200 should be considered candidates for pneumocystis (PCP) prophylaxis with trimethoprim/sulfamethoxazole, one double strength tablet daily or on alternate days. For those patients who cannot tolerate trimethoprim/sulfa, Dapsone 100mg twice weekly is an alternative. Other considerations for PCP prophylaxis would include atovaquone (Mepron®) 750mg daily, and monthly aerosolized or injectable pentamidine. Regimens which include trimethoprim/sulfamethoxazole or atovaquone may also be effective in preventing recurrent CNS toxoplasmosis.

Prophylaxis against disseminated mycobacterium avium complex infection is generally beneficial. This is indicated for patients with CD4 counts <100. The regimens include advanced macrolides such as Azithromycin 1,200mg weekly administered as two 600mg doses 12 hours apart, or daily clarithromycin 500mg twice daily.

Patients with CD4 <100 and underlying ocular cytomegalovirus (CMV) will benefit from long term suppressive therapy with IV ganciclovir or oral cytovene. Long term use of ganciclovir is often complicated by neutropenia while renal dysfunction may be caused by cytovene. The preservation of vision however, is an extremely important quality of life issue that must be decided individually.

The risks and benefits of prophylaxis should be weighed carefully. The ability of the patient to successfully ingest tablets or capsules must be considered among patients with advanced terminal illness. Clostridium difficile is much more likely to complicate antibiotic use in debilitated patients with carcinoma recently treated with chemotherapy. In select cases, withdrawal or curtailment of antibiotic prophylaxis may be beneficial.

Antiretrovirals

The most frequently used combinations of antiretroviral agents includes the nucleosides AZT 300mg every 12 hours, 3TC 150mg every 12 hours administered along with protease inhibitor most often Crixivan® 800mg every 8 hours. This regimen has been extremely effective in maintaining viral load level below the detectable levels for up to one year.

Patients placed on this regimen should be monitored initially at two weeks then monthly with a complete blood count and chemistries including amylase/lipase. Patients should have a baseline Vitamin B12 level and replacement therapy if indicated. Patients who receive Crixan should be well hydrated. Up to 10% of the patients receiving this agent may develop renal calculi. The protease inhibitors have also been noted to induce severe hyperglycemia in some patients.

At Calvary, patients with CD4 counts <500 who are alert and able to swallow are considered candidates for antiretroviral therapy. Although the long term prognosis for any given patient may be poor, the combination regimens are extremely effective. The regimen may be associated with an improved appetite and improvement in mentation. AZT alone was demonstrated to exert a beneficial effect on patients with AIDS/HIV related dementia.

It is essential that primary care physicians actively participate in the planning of therapeutic regimens for HIV infected patients with advanced cancer. The risks and benefits of each agent and or treatment modality must be carefully considered, discussed with the patient and when therapy is chosen it should be closely monitored. Comfort and quality of life should remain the most important concern.

References

1. Levine AM. Non-Hodgkin's lymphoma and other malignancies in AIDS. Semin Oncol 1987; 14 : 34-39.

2. Steinbrook R. Battling HIV on many fronts. New Eng Jr Med 1997; 337 : 779-781.

3. Fischl MA, Richman DD, Crieco MH, et al. The efficacy of azidothymidine (AZT) in the treatment of patients with AIDS and AIDS related complex. A double blind placebo controlled trial. New Eng Jr Med 1987; 317 : 185-189.

4. Savona S, Ohri A, Salloum E, Hewlett D. AIDS and malignancy: Experience in an inner city primary care hospital. Proc Ann Meet Am Soc Clin Oncol 1993; 12 : A.

5. Danzid JB, Brandt LJ, Reinus JF, Klein RS. Gastrointestinal malignancy in patients with AIDS. Am Jr Gastro 1991; 86 : 715-718.

UROLOGICAL CARE
Richard Bard

By the time a patient has been admitted to a palliative care facility all attempts at reversing (curing) the neoplastic process should have been exhausted. As a consequence, a realistic assessment of the patient's expected longevity should not exceed six months. The consideration to perform invasive procedures should keep this six month longevity period in mind as it would not be ethical to increase, even temporarily, a patient's morbidity unless his/her life span is projected to be long enough to justify any discomfort associated with continued therapy.

Catheter Care

Many hospitalized patients will have lost their ability to spontaneously evacuate their bladders and, as a consequence, will require "long-term" indwelling catheterization of the bladder. Increasing the success of catheterizing a patient can be achieved by first filling the barrel of a 10 cc syringe with KY jelly. The plunger is then placed back in the barrel and the jelly is injected into the urethra effectively creating a lubricated pathway for the Foley catheter. This procedure can minimize difficult catheterizations.

In catheterized patients, the urine will become colonized by gram negative bacteria within 24-48 hours in 100% of cases. However, only individuals who are symptomatic (febrile, chills, dysuria) should automatically receive antibiotic therapy. In non-symptomatic individuals, three methods of care can be utilized to prevent a clinical UTI or, in the worst case scenario, urosepsis. They are as follows:

Daily bladder irrigations until clear with 1/4% acetic acid solution to mechanically reduce the concentration of gram negative bacteria in the bladder.

Urinary acidification with an ascorbic acid 500 mg PO Q.I.D. to suppress microbial multiplication. Hipprex 1 gm BID or Mandelamine 500 mg Q.I.D. may also be used if the patient is able to swallow these medications.

Low dose antibacterial therapy (tri-weekly) therapy with a broad spectrum antibiotic such as trimethoprim may reduce microbial multiplication. Since resistant strains of bacteria may occur as a result of this regimen, it is essential that these agents not include an antibiotic which can be used for treatment of systemic infection if urosepsis should occur.

Bladder Spasm

Occasionally a patient with an indwelling Foley catheter will develop bladder spasms. This is the reaction of the bladder trying to expel a foreign body, i.e., the catheter. A first maneuver in such circumstances would be to deflate the balloon to 5cc's. If this does not help, rule out the possibility of malposition with the balloon being inflated in the urethra. If symptoms continue, propantheline bromide (Pro-Banthine®) 15 mg T.I.D. may be useful. Other antispasmodics such as diazepam (Valium®) and oxybutynin (Ditropan®) may be used if propantheline bromide (pro-Banthine®) is ineffective. One must also consider the known side effects of these medications which are xerostomia, tachycardia, ophthalmic symptoms and even sedation.

Care of Nephrostomy Tubes

Since the advent of sonographically placed nephrostomy tubes, i.e. percutaneous nephrostomy, the need for open renal surgery for nephrostomy placement has become a thing of the past. However, these smaller diameter tubes require considerable attention which includes cleansing and dressing of the skin site daily. Frequently these tubes become obstructed and require irrigation with normal saline under high pressure via a 5cc syringe.

When percutaneously placed tubes cannot be unobstructed or become dislodged in a terminal patient, the dilemma of what clinical course to pursue becomes self-evident. Blocked nephrostomy tubes which require replacement under sonographic control entail movement of the patient to a radiology suite as well as physical manipulation and could result in renal hemorrhage or urosepsis.

Thus, the physician must decide if such risks are justified, and weigh them against the patient's overall clinical status and expected length of survival.

In the case of a dislodged nephrostomy tube, attempts can be made within two hours of discovery to place a small Foley catheter (10 or 12 French) down the *hopefully* still patent nephrostomy tract into the renal pelvis. If this is successful, the patient is spared a potential surgical procedure. However, failing to replace the dislodged tube presents the same aforementioned dilemma of whether to subject the patient to the sonographic replacement of a non-functioning nephrostomy tube.

Dermatologic Conditions of the Genitalia

Although there are a multitude of cutaneous conditions that affect the genitalia, only a few are significant in the palliative setting.

Candidiasis - Manifests itself as characteristic confluent erythematous areas on the scrotum, groin, and penis. Most often this is successfully treated by control of the patients diabetes mellitus (if present) and use of Lotrimin cream which is antifungal. Systemic antimycotic agents should not, in general, be used for isolated cutaneous problems.

Herpes Progenitalis - Vesicals having an erythematous base which then slough leaving a denuded lesion are characteristic of this entity. They can occur on the labia, scrotum, or penis. The designated therapy is Zovirax® (acyclovir) ointment applied topically to the lesions T.I.D. as well as oral administration (800 mg po 4-5x/day x 5-6 days). This generally results in rapid crusting, involution, and healing of the cutaneous eruption.

Pyogenic Cutaneous Lesions - Although relatively uncommon, these lesions should be diagnosed by culture and then treated with a broad spectrum, oral antibiotic and/or topical triple antibiotic ointment T.I.D.

Other Infectious Conditions

There may be a rare instance of non-obstructive pyelonephritis or epididymitis with or without involvement of the testes (epididymo-orchitis). Depending on severity, these conditions can be successfully treated with oral or intravenous antibiotic therapy as well as local therapy (heat in the form of warm soaks) to the gonad in the later condition.

Emergency (Surgical) Urological Conditions

There are a few situations at Calvary Hospital which may require surgical intervention in which a urological consultation is in order.

Paraphimosis - Inability to reduce the foreskin over the glans penis is painful and may result in gangrene of the paraphimosis tissue. Thus, it is imperative, if initial attempts at reduction are unsuccessful, to obtain a urological consultation.

Obstruction of Ureter Resulting in Azotemia - A significant number of patients with pelvic neoplasm (prostate, cervix, rectum) will have obstruction of the distal ureters resulting in progressive obstruction of the upper urinary tracts. Unless a patient is unusually robust with a projected life span of greater than six months, percutaneous placement of nephrostomy tubes should be avoided. If percutaneous nephrostomy is performed in the more robust patient, it should be done with a view towards replacing the nephrostomy tube with an internal ureteral stent. Once internal ureteral stenting has been accomplished, the patient can be considered for an alternate level of care such as discharge home with paramedical aid or to a nursing facility.

Testicular or Scrotal Abscess - Surgical drainage and antibiotic therapy are mandatory within a brief time framework in order to avoid clinical sepsis. If cutaneous scrotal gangrene occurs (Fournier's Gangrene), wide debridement of the gangrenous tissue by a urologist should be performed, either under local anesthesia at the bedside or in a hospital setting.

Meatal Stenosis - This problem will be discovered at the time of attempted urethral (bladder) catheterization. The meatal stricture will require dilatation before catheterization can be accomplished and, as a consequence, a urological consultation is required.

Attention to preventing or expeditiously caring for the aforementioned problems can add immeasurably to a patient's comfort.

CARDIOVASCULAR PROBLEMS
Sharad Jaitly

The occurrence of cardiac problems increases with age in any given population. We also know that the occurrence of cancer increases with age. Therefore, it is not uncommon to find cardiac problems in our institution.

Cardiovascular abnormalities are being diagnosed at an earlier stage and it is not unusual to find hematologist/oncologists consulting with cardiologists regarding clinical problems. Problems related to heart failure, pericardial effusion, cardiac arrhythmias and ischemic heart disease often occur. Sometimes, anemia-related symptoms and not uncommon findings suggestive of endocarditis or new onset of heart murmurs are other interesting aspects of cardiac problems that physicians must consider.

These are the commonest causes for consultation. Treatment will be discussed in relation to palliative care in the setting of terminal illness.

Arrhythmias

Arrhythmias that occur unrelated to the history of cancer have prevalence similar to what one might expect in the non-cancer population. On the other hand arrhythmias directly related to cancer per se are an interesting entity. Every cancer related arrhythmia is seen in association with metastatic disease to the pericardium, myocardium or endocardium. The heart is the site of the metastatic disease when the primary is melanoma, breast, lung or lymphoma. Certain leukemias involve myocardium or endocardium as well and present as infiltrates that are clearly seen on echocardiography or at autopsies. The pericardial and myocardial lesions can also be detected by echocardiography. Incidence of cardiac metastases is perhaps increasing as survival pattern and means of detection are improving.

Clinical manifestations of arrhythmias vary from chest pain, angina, dyspnea, heart failure, palpitations, and dizziness. Sometimes nonspecific nausea or even fatigue can be the only symptom of presentation.

Tachyarrhythmias

Tachyarrhythmias, both supraventricular and ventricular, are of great importance in detection as well as comfort management. Among tachyarrhythmias, supraventricular tachycardia (SVT) or proximal atrial tachycardia (PAT), atrial flutter and atrial fibrillation are the commonest arrhythmias seen in this population. Supraventricular tachycardias are managed on the basis of hemodynamic instability. In the conventional setting (without the terminal illness), adenosine or electric shock are the therapeutic modalities of choice. These are followed by verapamil, digoxin or beta blockers intravenously. Once the patient is stabilized, oral medications may be used.

A palliative approach on the other hand, would consist of adenosine as the drug of choice. Electrical shock is not employed at our institution. The advantage of using adenosine in the setting of palliative care for supraventricular tachycardia treatment is two fold. First, it is instantaneous in its action. An SVT can be converted to a normal sinus rhythm with the use of bolus adenosine 80-90% of the time. Twelve mg of adenosine is given via a large anticubital vein. Secondly, patient tolerance is excellent because there are minimal side effects. Verapamil, digoxin and beta blockers are generally used only in patients who have converted to normal sinus rhythm, are stabilized hemodynamically and who have reasonable survival prognosis.

Relatively uncommon but felt to be very unstable is atrial flutter. Patients are digitalized and type 1A drugs such as procainamide or quinidine are commonly employed to keep the ventricular rate under control and/or to keep patients in stable rhythm. On the other hand, in a conventional setting in a non-cancer type of patient, one would employ electrical cardioversion as the procedure of choice. Anticoagulation remains controversial, but may be used if survival is expectantly more than six weeks, and if the ventricular rate is controlled with digitalis, a calcium blocker or a beta-blocker.

Treatment for atrial fibrillation is similar to atrial flutter. In a conventional non-palliative setting, cardioversion is attempted in new onset variety. Control of ventricular rate and therapeutic anticoagulation are the major goals in the chronic variety. Treatment in the palliative setting is to stabilize ventriclular rate and attempt to convert by using digitalis and type 1A drugs. Anticoagulation is used only if survival is expectantly at least six weeks and must be discussed with the patient and family prior to making such a commitment.

Frequent VPC's and Non-sustained Ventricular Tachycardia (NSVT)

VPC's are commonly seen on a routine EKG. The recommendation to treat frequent occurrences of non-sustained VTs with suitable antiarrhythmic drugs like procainamide or beta blockers should be made only if survival is expectantly weeks to months. It is recommended to follow N-acetyl procainamide (NAPA) and procainamide blood levels. It is also important to follow liver and kidney functions in these patients. In a conventional approach, cardioversion is often the procedure of choice but is not indicated in the palliative setting.

Bradyarrhythmias

The most common bradyarrhythmias are sick sinus syndrome, second degree AV Block and very rarely, AV dissociation. Conventional approach to any of the bradyarrhythmias is a pacemaker. A patient's capacity for exercise or physical activity is another determinant. Atropine intravenously is usually recommended for our patients. In a palliative setting, a patient's expected survival is always a major consideration.

Heart Failure

In the setting of terminal cancer, heart failure is commonly seen as a result of severe anemia, anthracycline cardiac toxicity, acute pulmonary embolism or hypertensive and atherosclerotic heart disease. It is important to distinguish between diastolic and systolic heart failure. The presence or absence of cardiomegaly and specific findings on echo, can distinguish between the two and appropriate therapy recommended.

Treatment in this setting is directed toward respiratory distress, peripheral and pulmonary edema. Use of morphine intravenously or subcutaneously is of a therapeutic benefit in reducing the symptoms and improving the hemodynamics of a failing heart. Supplemental oxygenation, use of diuretics, judicious use of angiotensin converting enzyme (ACE) inhibitors and close follow up of electrolytes and renal function can improve the symptoms dramatically in many of these patients. Use of bronchodilators in the presence of pulmonary edema are recommended only if wheezing is a predominant feature. Arrhythmia correction with suitable agents is used adjuvantly depending upon patients tolerance. Use of nitrates as topical patches are excellent when angina or ischemic heart disease coexists. Transfusions in patients with short survival prognosis is generally not recommended. However, it may be very useful where reasonably good functional capacity or outcome is anticipated, for instance if a patient may return home for a few weeks or be transferred to a nursing home. Patients must then be observed very closely and the use of diuretics may be necessary during and after the completion of the transfusion. Conventional therapy including digoxin, nitrates and ACE inhibitors should be continued on a routine basis as long as a patient can tolerate them . Food restriction and salt restriction must be done modestly as patients in a palliative setting are usually anorectic and we do not wish to remove any comfort they may derive from a preferred food.

Ischemic heart disease

Angina, acute coronary insufficiency or myocardial infarction can occur in the setting of terminally ill patients. Invariably, symptoms are not overtly exhibited by the patients. Silent ischemia and silent myocardial infarctions are common in the elderly population and may also occur in advanced cancer patients. Lack of physical stress and poor functional status limit the detection of angina in many of these patients. The role of nitrates topically or sublingually is indicated. Nitrates may be used with calcium blockers and beta blockers especially in the presence of coexistent hypertension. Buffered aspirin is generally not used in these patients. There is an increased risk of inducing bleeding because of coexisting abnormalities such as coagulopathy, peptic ulcer disease or abnormal platelet function. Acute coronary syndromes including coronary insufficiency, unstable angina or myocardial infarction are rarely encountered, but if they occur they are also treated with nitrates, morphine, oxygen and possibly beta or calcium blockers. Morphine plays a major role in comforting patients who have cardiac pain or dyspnea.

Endocarditis

Endocarditis of non-bacterial thrombotic, marantic and bacterial etiologies in the setting of advanced cancer patients can occur. If a patient has new onset or changing heart murmurs during the setting of prolonged febrile episodes, with no other evidence of infection or sepsis, endocarditis should be suspected. Diagnostic studies and treatment are based on expected survival in these patients. Antibiotics given intravenously for at least four to six weeks may not be practical nor even indicated in this setting.

Pulmonary embolism and peripheral venous thrombosis

Pulmonary embolism should be suspected if the patient has a sudden cardiorespiratory deterioration with a fall in blood pressure, severe acute onset of dyspnea, diaphoresis, cyanosis and tachycardia. Frequently the lungs are clear to auscultation. Diagnosis is made on clinical and electrocardiographic findings. Ventilation-perfusion (VQ) scans are usually inappropriate in the palliative care setting. Treatment consists of oxygenation and morphine to alleviate symptoms of anxiety as well as dyspnea. Use of diuretics in the setting of pulmonary congestion is helpful. Intravenous anticoagulation with heparin and the use of thrombolytic agents are rarely indicated.

Acute Arterial Occlusion

Acute arterial occlusion is a rare yet devastating complication which may occur even in the final weeks of life. The occlusion sites most often seen at Calvary Hospital are the common femoral artery and more peripherally the popliteal artery.

Conservative therapy even with anticoagulation and other supportive measures invariably leads to severe debilitation, pain, and gangrenous necrosis of the affected limb. As soon as a diagnosis is suspected, active interventional therapy is undertaken to avoid the grave consequences of occlusion of the circulation to the affected limb.

Doppler studies with subsequent invasive procedures are done to establish arterial integrity. Despite a palliative setting, aggressive therapy is almost always indicated.

Peripheral arterial occlusion is an exceptionally rare occurrence at Calvary Hospital. An acute thrombotic episode or an embolus are the mechanisms leading to acute arterial insufficiency. Severe pain and loss of function leading to gangrenous necrosis of the affected limb may be seen.

Acute intervention is taken only if the morbidity from the arterial occlusion is going to be overwhelming. Keeping in mind that any intervention planned to reduce or minimize the suffering or morbidity from such an event must be discussed with the patient and the family. The issue of undertaking an aggressive approach (with palliation in mind) should be carefully evaluated. Investigative procedures such as a Doppler study or an angiogram are part of this evaluation before the patient is referred for diagnostic studies.

An aggressive approach in such a circumstance is rarely undertaken in the palliative care setting.

Conclusion

The treatment modalities in the setting of the terminally ill patient is mainly palliative and directed towards the relief of symptoms. The goal is to reduce dyspnea, anxiety and pain. Supplemental oxygen alone may control symptoms especially if oxygen saturation is known to be compromised. The judicious use of cardiac drugs may be beneficial. Aggressive therapies like cardioversion, thrombolytic therapy, blood transfusions, anticoagulation or the use of pressors is rarely recommended in this setting of palliative care. If the physician takes the time to discuss issues and goals of palliative treatment, the patients and families rarely disagree with this approach.

References

1. Braunwald E. A Textbook of Cardiovascular Medicine. Heart disease. Philadelphia: W.B.Saunders, 5th ed. 1997.

2. Adenosine vs. verapamil in the treatment of supra ventricular tachycardia: A randomized double-crossover trial. Am Heart J 1992;123: pp 1543.

3. Quality of life among 5025 patients with left ventricular dysfunction randomized placebo and evalopril. J Am Coll Cardiology 1994; 23: pp 393.

CPR AND DNR
Gail Chrzanowski

How aggressive medical care should be as the patient's physical status is declining is a joint decision that must be shared by the patient, the family or health care proxy, and the physician. The decision to perform Cardio-pulmonary resuscitation (CPR) is a choice that must be decided upon in the palliative care setting. This is particularly important when a patient's condition is changing rapidly. Cardio-pulmonary resuscitation can include external compressions upon a patient's chest to foster circulation, performing artificial breathing, possibly intubating the patient and connecting a patient to a respirator.

Starting in the late 1950's, cardio-pulmonary resuscitation was used primarily to restore life to previously healthy individuals who had experienced cardiac or respiratory arrest during surgery or as a result of drowning, electrical shock, acute myocardial infarction or a cardiac arrhythmia.

Today CPR is tried on almost every person who suffers a cardiac or respiratory event. CPR is seen as emergency treatment and therefore, consent to perform CPR is presumed. The victim is incapable of stating what he wants done and if care is not given immediately the person will die.[1]

The use of CPR in terminally ill cancer patients is problematic. It provides little chance of survival and perhaps is used too aggressively. Numerous studies have been done to determine outcomes of CPR in various groups.[2,3,4,5,6] In 1983, Bidell et al. published a study of 294 patients resuscitated in a Boston Hospital.[4] None of the patients with metastatic cancer survived until discharge. The most common diagnosis of the 294 patients was coronary artery disease. Twenty percent (59 people) had a history of cancer and of the 59 patients with cancer only 4 (7%) survived resuscitation. However, not one of these four was discharged alive from the hospital. It was felt that none survived because of the multi-organ system failure associated with cancer. The patient's performance status prior to hospitalization was also important in predicting the results of the cardiopulmonary resuscitation. Severely debilitated patients did not do well.

The duration of the arrest also plays an important part in the success of the resuscitation. In one study, patients who were resuscitated and were alert and did not require pressors 24 hours after the event had a survival rate of 35%. Only 9% of the patients survived to discharge when CPR attempts were longer than fifteen minutes.[6]

CPR or the decision not to resuscitate (DNR) should be discussed and agreed upon by the patient, physician and family or health care proxy early in the hospital stay. Physicians are responsible for the quality of information given to the patient and family so that a plan of care may be instituted. The doctor must inform the patient of the vulnerability of the patient during CPR, of the success rate, of the post arrest consequences and post resuscitation functional status so that the patient or family may make an informed decision.

Many patients with terminal disease have formulated living wills or have requested Do Not Resuscitate (DNR) orders. If such an advanced directive is unknown or when in doubt, resuscitation will prevail. Since 1976, in New York State a physician may write an order to withhold CPR.[7] Currently, a patient and or surrogate must be notified if a DNR order is written.

It is the patient's right to forgo medical treatment.[8] The patient decides whether or not CPR is to be withheld. If the patient does not want to be resuscitated a DNR order should be written. If the patient is too ill to express specific or otherwise incapacitated then the decision to forgo resuscitation can be made by the surrogate decision maker or health care proxy.[9]

At times the patient's right to autonomy is juxtaposed to the idea of futility. A physician is not ethically obligated to make a specific diagnostic or therapeutic procedure available to a patient even on request if the use of such a procedure would be futile.[10] However, futility is often vague. The goal must be clearly defined. For example, is resuscitation successful if the patient's pulse returns and must be placed on a respirator and will not recover once life support is discontinued?

For a patient to be autonomous, the patient chooses from the available treatment alternatives that are appropriate for his condition. The success of CPR is judged by the attending physician by its ability to benefit the patient in a manner that is viewed as appropriate by both the patient and the attending physician.

Fabre-Langendoen reevaluated the goals of medicine citing the Hippocratic Oath. "To cure sometimes to relieve often, to comfort always."[8,11] The American College of Physicians further reiterates the same aims, "to prevent disease, restore health and provide palliation and comfort for those diseases that can not be cured."[11] None of the concepts of medicine is to squeeze out the last few breaths of life. Physicians must communicate with their patients, inform patients of goals and outcomes, respect a patient's autonomy, but not offer therapies that do not benefit.

A physician should stress all the comfort measures that would be available at the time of imminent death so that a patient can be reassured that he will not suffer. These measures may include oxygen, pain medication, morphine to help breathing, suctioning if necessary, anti-anxiety medications and a great deal of emotional support. A well informed patient that communicates with a compassionate physician has little disagreement in deciding futility of medical care. At Calvary Hospital, 99.9% have a DNR order in place before death occurs.

References

1. Emergency cardiac care committee and subcommittees of the AHA Guidelines for CPR. Part VII. Ethical considerations in resuscitation. JAMA 1992;268: pp 2282-88.

2. Arena FP, Perlin M, Turnbull AD. Initial experiences with a code-no code resuscitation system in cancer patients. Crit Care Med 1980;8: pp 788-89.

3. Hershey CO, Fisher L. Why outcome of cardiopulmonary resuscitation in general wads is poor. Lancet 1982;1: pp 31-34.

4. Bisdell SE, Delbance TL, Cook EF, Epstein TH. Survival after cardiopulmonary resuscitation in the hospital. N Engl J Med 1983;309: pp 569-76.

5. Sowden GR, Robins DW, Boshett PF. Factors associated with survival and eventual status following cardiac arrest. Anesthesia 1984;39: pp 39-46.

6. Rosenbaum EA, Shenkman L. Predicting outcome of in hospital cardiopulmonary resuscitation. Crit Care Med 1988;16: pp 583-86.

7. Swenson E, Matsiura J, Martinson IN. Effects of resuscitation for patients with metastatic cancers and chronic heart disease. News Res 1979;28: pp 151-53.

8. Fabre-Langendoen K. Resuscitation of patients with metastatic cancer. Is transient benefit still futile? Arch Int Med 1991;151: pp 235-39.

9. President's Commission for the Study of Ethical Problems in Medicine and Biomedical and Behavioral Research. Deciding to forgo life-sustaining treatment. Washington, DC: Gov Print Off 1983; pp 534.

10. Council on Ethical and Judicial Affairs. Guidelines for the appropriate use of do-not-resuscitate orders. Chicago: American Medical Association, 1990.

11. American College of Physicians Ethics Committee. American College of Physician Ethics Committee Manual 1. Ann Int Med 1989; pp 111-247.

CALVARY HOSPITAL BLOOD TRANSFUSION PRACTICES
Cynthia Collins and Michael J. Brescia

Calvary Hospital has implemented blood transfusion practices based on recent changes in the national guidelines and has also studied blood transfusion practice in advanced cancer patients.

Calvary's patients are more difficult to assess regarding the need for transfusion. Many symptoms related to low hemoglobin and low hematocrit could also be attributed to advanced disease, previous cancer treatment, and/or high doses of opiates used for the palliation of pain. Many of Calvary's patients are admitted directly after active chemotherapy and/or radiation therapy and a blood transfusion may be necessary. Other patients have underlying anemia related to their disease process and/or previous treatment. Still, other patients may require transfusion as palliation for symptoms related to advanced hematological disease.

Calvary Hospital conducted a retrospective review of thirty transfusion events in 1995. The objectives of the study were to determine why end stage cancer patients are transfused at Calvary Hospital in a palliative care setting. Before the 1995 study, Calvary's criteria for transfusions were based on the American College of Pathologist's (ACP) guidelines. The ACP guidelines suggest that patients should be transfused only if they have symptoms related to a reduced oxygen-carrying capacity of the blood, despite the hemoglobin level. Normovolemic patients should experience syncope, dyspnea, tachycardia, angina, postural hypotension, or transient ischemic attack before red blood cells are transfused. Also included are non-symptomatic patients who are actively bleeding who experience a drop in hematocrit of 6% or more in a twenty-four hour period and patients with a history of cerebrovascular disease.

Thirty transfusion events were reviewed, objective clinical data were obtained. Calvary Hospital has shown a decline in the number of patients transfused over the past few years. In 1993, 140 patients were transfused, in 1994, 106, and in 1995, 98 patients were transfused. In 1993, 2,083 patients were admitted to Calvary, in 1994, 2,240 and in 1995, 2,433. The number of transfusions at Calvary is relatively small; only 4% of Calvary's entire patient population received blood transfusions in 1995 compared with 6.7% in 1994, and 4.3% in 1993.

Calvary's physicians were interviewed by a registered nurse to learn if there were other indicators for transfusion that were more specific to end-stage cancer patients. It was discovered that acute care guidelines are not always appropriate in the palliative care setting. Calvary Hospital's blood transfusion criteria are now based on the 1995 transfusion study. New criteria were added to those existing. Some new findings concluded that automatic, numerical transfusions triggers should be avoided. Packed red blood cells should be transfused on a unit-by-unit basis, with clinical evaluation of the patient's response to each transfusion and erythropoietin therapy considered when appropriate. Patients should be transfused based on active symptoms related to a low hemoglobin and hematocrit.

Discussion

Objective indicators such as vital signs may be influenced by pain and the use of opiates in pain palliation and/or decreased mobility. Vital signs may not always be accurate indicators even when there is sustained chronic bleeding, i.e., hematuria, vaginal, and rectal bleeding. There may be several reasons why vital signs are maintained. Physiologic adaption to anemia is well documented and another factor may be prolonged bed rest. Dyspnea as an indicator may also be attributed to advanced processes, pain, metabolic changes, and/or comorbid conditions and may also be masked by opiates and bed rest. Syncope, postural, hypotension and transient ischemic attacks (TIA) were not reported as a symptoms in the study. Calvary's patients may instead complain of dizziness, profound weakness, experience a change in mental status or have a decrease in mobility or functional status. Calvary physicians may also transfuse patients if there is a request from the patient or family in the presence of active bleeding which is causing extreme psychological distress.

The majority of patients at Calvary received two units of blood per single order, compared to ACP guidelines to transfuse on a unit-by-unit basis. Calvary physicians prefer to transfuse two units per single order due to poor venous access and patient comfort. The quality of life and kind of complicated disease require the physician to make a subjective decision when ordering a blood transfusion.

After reviewing the results of the study, new criteria for transfusion were added and implemented:

To stabilize patient for discharge home or to another facility;

To maintain patient's ability to ambulate;

To maintain patient's ability to perform activities of daily living;

Altered mental status related to anemia;

Increased weakness, dizziness, and/or profound fatigue;

Rapid drop in hematocrit 4-5% in 24-48 hours with symptomatic changes in patient;

Active bleeding (acute, chronic, physiologic);

Cardiac symptoms related to anemia;

Psychological (patient/family request) such as fear of exsanguination;

Anemia which causes or aggravates heart failure;

Prolong life until a grieving/distraught relative can reach the bedside from a distant location;

For dyspnea, associated with physiologic deprivation of diminished oxygen carrying blood due to anemia. Requires confirmation and documentation, accurate respiratory assessment and/or use of pulse oximeter and past medical history.

Palliative care for terminal cancer patients at Calvary Hospital is an essential part of the final stage of life. Calvary's patients are unique and may not always fit into established standards of care as depicted in the Island Peer Review Organization study and/or acute health care management guidelines utilized by third party payers. It is difficult to identify specific guidelines for what is appropriate for every individual at the end of life and his or her response to the dying process. Despite these extended criteria for blood usage, the actual utilization of blood transfusion is quite low at Calvary Hospital.

References

1. Gleeson C. Blood transfusion and its benefits in palliative care. Palliat Med 1995;9: pp 307--13.

2. Welch G. Prudent strategies for elective red blood cell transfusion. Ann Med, 1992; 116: pp 393-402.

3. Pickett G. Red blood cell transfusion practices in New York. IPRO Quality Improvement Study, 1995.

PHYSICAL THERAPY
Edward Casey

In 1971, the National Cancer Program of the National Cancer Institute established seven key objectives for improving the care of cancer patients. The seventh was "Develop the means to improve the rehabilitation of cancer patients." The means or disciplines recommended to attain this totally integrated rehabilitation are: physician, nurse, chaplain, physical therapist, occupational therapist, social service worker, psychiatrist, speech and hearing therapists, prosthodontist, prosthetist/orthotist and vocational counselor.

The consequences of both the cancer and the treatment that our patients undergo, create a wide variety of disabilities with corresponding rehabilitation needs. Physical therapy is only one discipline in the total integrated rehabilitation caring of the cancer disabled population at Calvary Hospital.

The physical therapy activity at Calvary is offered to a patient population with progressive disease, increasing disability and decreasing function, who are being cared for in a palliative care setting. Classification of each patient's potential is essential. The patient must be evaluated for expected response in the categories of restorative, supportive and palliative types of treatment.

The physical therapy staff is comprised of three part time physical therapists and a full time physiatrist. Each patient referred is initially evaluated by the physiatrist and depending upon the patient's clinical cognitive status, a decision on active physical therapy is determined at that time. Patients referred remain on the physiatrist census until disposition, i.e., discharge home, nursing home, hospital, or death. A patient is followed by the physiatrist whether or not he/she is active in the physical therapy program. If a patient is referred to the physical therapist and then deteriorates clinically, the patient is discharged from active physical therapy but followed by the physiatrist. If that patient again becomes clinically capable of partaking in a physical therapy program, he/she is resumed without need for another consult request from the attending physician. This has allowed patients to be active when clinically and functionally capable, to recuperate when in the dynamic low trough and then resume when willing and able.

The transporting of patients from their individual rooms via wheelchair or stretcher on elevators to a physical therapy unit and returning proved to be unrealistic for most patients. Therefore, the bedside, in room and corridor ambulation became the standard practice.

At the bedside both active and assisted range of motion is initiated only after bone status is determined. Rolling side to side, changing position from supine to sitting, and use of upper extremity to aid position change are progressively introduced. Sitting balance, ruling out postural hypotension and base line pulse rate precede attempt to stand. Standing with contact guard, walking in place and then walking shuffle or reciprocal gait follows. Increasing the distance ambulated and use of a walker or cane is dependent upon the individual's capability and need. In the patient's room at bed level, manual resistive exercises may again be introduced after determining bone status. A restorator offering reciprocal bilateral lower extremity exercise at conventional chair height can be used for aerobic stimulation. Resistance is altered for each patient and vital signs are maintained. Active range of motion of upper extremities with deep inspiration at shoulder flexion and expiration when arms are returned to the side promote good pulmonary exchange.

The Physical Therapy Department also recommends activity for Calvary Outpatients and Calvary Home Care patients. Orthoses and prostheses have been prescribed and used functionally by cancer disabled individuals. These orthoses have been Sterno Occipital Mandibular Immobilizer (SOMI) and thoracic lumbar braces to stabilize areas of vertebral metastases. Humeral and femoral fracture cast braces have also been employed.

Cancer is not always the problem. One patient with prostate cancer and no apparent bone metastases who developed a peripheral vascular problem required amputation. A below knee temporary prosthesis and then a permanent prosthesis were prescribed and he is now ambulating functionally.

If only supportive care is the goal and the prognosis is limited with expectation of continuing disease and disability, every effort should be made to avoid the secondary effects of prolonged bed rest and prolonged incapacity. The group in the restorative category without remarkable residual disability requires the greatest use of the rehabilitation team up to and including Social Service and vocational planning, retraining and guidance groups.

While the prognosis of the patient must be considered, it should not be the determining factor as to the amount of treatment to be given. Total debility and chronic pain will affect any attempt at functional recovery. However, palliation in itself, can be a justifiable goal of a rehabilitation program.

References

1. Papers presented at the 15th Annual Clinical Conference on Cancer. Rehabilitation of the cancer patient. University of Texas, Houston, Texas. Year Book Medical Publishers, Inc., 1970.

2. Objective - National Cancer Program. Develop the means to improve the rehabilitation of cancer patients. Department of Health Education and Welfare Publication (NIH) 74-590.

3. Dietz, JH. Rehabilitation Oncology. New York: John Wiley & Sons, 1981.

4. Marcant D, Rapin CH. Role of the physiotherapist in palliative car. J Pain Sympt Manag. 1993;8: pp 220-25.

5. American Cancer Society. Rehabilitation and Supportive Care of the Cancer Patient. In: Textbook of Clinical Oncology, 2nd edition.

DIAGNOSTIC RADIOLOGY
Arnold Berrett

Radiology in advanced cancer patients presents multiple challenges. It is extremely important to keep the X-ray examination brief and simple. The goal is to obtain the maximum information in the shortest possible time with the least inconvenience. The three areas of concentration in radiology are the chest, abdomen, and bones.

Chest

An examination of the chest is obtained on most patients shortly after admission. Since Calvary patients are seriously ill, some physicians may request an examination using the portable apparatus. The diagnostic quality of portable X-rays is generally not satisfactory and we discourage use of this method. Every attempt is made to transport the patient to the X-ray Department. There may only be a single opportunity to study the patient and, therefore we try to obtain as much information as possible at that time.

A frequent finding is an inflammatory process in the chest superimposed upon a known carcinoma of the lung. When these patients are treated with antibiotics a follow-up examination performed after a short interval of time is usually unproductive. As a general rule, the patient's clinical improvement takes place before the resolution of the inflammatory process is manifest on the X-ray. Under these circumstances it is appropriate to delay ordering a repeat examination to assess the degree of resolution.

A finding which sometimes causes confusion is diminished air entry at the bases of the lung. This finding usually indicates the presence of fluid in the pleural cavity. There are other conditions which may produce a similar picture. At Calvary Hospital a common cause is intraabdominal disease. Under these circumstances the domes of the diaphragm are elevated.

When disease is advanced, there is usually evidence of metastatic disease in the bony thorax on the chest examination. If the lesions are small, interpretation is very difficult. Radiographic examination of the ribs is of only limited value in this setting. The reason for this is twofold. The ribs are curved structures almost semicircular, and do not lend themselves easily to evaluation by conventional X-rays. Secondly, the anterior ends of the ribs are not bony, but are made of cartilage which cannot be demonstrated with conventional X-rays.

Abdomen

Examination of the abdomen can present a challenge. Determining whether or not there is obstruction in the gastrointestinal tract is sometimes difficult because of wide spread intraabdominal disease. X-rays taken with the patient erect should only be considered if perforation is suspected. Under these circumstances a radiograph of the chest is obtained with the patient in a sitting position. In order to include the diaphragms and the upper abdomen the film is moved downwards thus making it possible to determine whether or not there is an accumulation of air under the domes of the diaphragm. When ascites is encountered, interpretation of abdominal studies is further complicated by the obscuration by the fluid. Procedures using barium are restricted since patients are rarely able to participate properly.

Bones

The study of the bones is a very important area of concentration. Prior to undertaking the evaluation of metastatic disease, it is necessary to consider the characteristics of osteoporosis. First, the overall status of the skeleton should be reviewed. In the presence of severe osteoporosis, osteolytic metastatic disease portends an unfavorable outcome. On the other hand, if the skeleton is normal prior to the development of the malignant process, the outcome is likely to be more favorable. Such a patient will usually have less pain, a lower incidence of pathological fractures, and weight bearing may be possible.

In the presence of severe osteoporosis, metastatic disease can be difficult to diagnose. Incidentally, when the bony architecture is disturbed by associated degenerative disease, small metastatic foci may be obscure.

One special type of osteoporosis is disuse osteoporosis. This is a localized condition usually found in an immobilized limb. When an arm or leg is immobilized, loss of bone takes place at a rapid rate. If this is prolonged, the bones become ghost-like in appearance on X-ray. Fractures, osteomyelitis and metastatic deposits can be very difficult to diagnose with any degree of certainty in the presence of disuse osteoporosis.

Comprehensive evaluation of bones is necessary before making definitive decisions about weight bearing and nursing care, as well as quality of life issues.

The exact location of pain influences the decision as to the type of X-ray examination to be performed. For example, if the patient is experiencing pain in the region of the humerus, this can easily be examined for tenderness by local palpation. On the other hand, the hip joint is surrounded by extensive soft tissue structures. Palpation of the area is limited, making it difficult to identify the exact location of the disease. This situation calls for a more extensive X-ray examination. A suspected pathological fracture of the neck of the femur may not be the cause of a patient's pain, but rather a lesion in the nearby pelvic bones. Thus, if a restricted examination of the hip is undertaken, an obvious lesion may be overlooked.

Special Procedures

In certain situations, we refer our patients to a nearby facility for a radioactive bone scan. Keep in mind that although this study is very sensitive, it is a non-specific examination. Even in patients with known cancer, the bone scan may be positive as a result of infection or trauma. Patients with suspected intracranial disease can also be referred for CAT or MRI examination. Generally, no diagnostic studies should be undertaken if there is no intention to act on the study.

THEORY AND PHILOSOPHY AND THE CANCER CARE TECHNICIAN PROGRAM
Patricia Tennell

Theory and Philosophy

The nurses of Calvary Hospital believe that compassionate nursing care, offered with sensitivity and competence, is essential to a good quality of life for patients and their families. Empowering of the patients is of prime importance and is manifest in the belief that the patient has the right to decide what persons constitute family. This approach helps the patient to retain as much control as possible as well as empowering the family members. Our mission is multi-fold: 1) to help patients and their families cope with terminal illness; 2) to offer physical, spiritual and psychological comfort; 3) to ensure that the patient's dignity is maintained; 4) to allow patients and families to retain their decision making authority. The nursing team is comprised of cancer care technicians, nurses' aides, licensed practical nurses, and registered nurses whose contributions are invaluable. The professional nurse's role offers opportunities for independent practice. Nurse specialists provide sophisticated nursing practices that include ostomy specialists, intravenous therapy nurses and an infection control nurse.

The areas typically addressed by the nursing team include physical, psychosocial and spiritual. These problems are often interrelated. The physical problems are usually due to pain, mobility, ventilation, nutrition and hydration, skin integrity, elimination, self-care, and protection from infection and physical hazards.

In delivering physical care, symptom control is paramount. The nurse's role is to reduce suffering. For example, a simple measure such as offering nutrition in small frequent feedings rather than large meals may make a difference to the anorectic patient. Another example is the relieving of dyspnea which may not only improve the body's physiology but also contribute to the relief of patient anxiety. Pain control is central but not without its complications. Sometimes the challenge is to strike a balance between pain control and the level of cognition desired by the patient or the family. Ultimately, the patient's choice is usually respected and it is what the patient believes as appropriate.

The areas that are usually labeled as psychosocial include impaired communications, altered sensory perception, impaired thought process, anxiety, inability to cope, disturbed self-concept, potential for self-harm, inhibited expression of grief and bereavement, and thwarted development achievement. Patients have different life experiences and consequently are at different levels of coping with their disease. Some patients never achieve a level of acceptance of their disease and its likely consequences. Family members share these concerns as well and exhibit different mechanisms.

Sometimes our task is complicated by the fact that the needs of the patient and the family member conflict. We are aware that the stress of death may bring to the surface both overt and latent problems in family dynamics. In each case, we try to guide the patients toward resolution of such differences. No matter how complex the dynamic is, the needs of patients and their families are never abandoned.

Nurses also provide spiritual support as spiritual nurturing relates to the values of the patient's life. Our staff appreciates the patient's individual notion of spirituality, and does not substitute its own values. Nurses maintain their own belief systems, but patients are never deprived nor influenced against their own spiritual supports.

The patient and family are offered hope, helpful education, problem solving, and realistic grounding when unrealistic beliefs are apparent. Our hope is that patients perceive themselves to be in control rather than dependent on a system that leaves them helpless.

A sense of normality in the patient's life is predicated on perceiving it as a continuum. Contacts with all significant others, grandchildren, friends and even pets is encouraged. Special occasions such as birthdays, anniversaries and other important events are respected and celebrated. The community of patients, family and staff also acknowledge the usual holidays with activities and entertainment for those who are well enough to attend. Calvary is viewed as the place where the patient lives, not merely as a place to be housed.

Nurses recognize that support must be provided for families while engaged in the letting go process and in their course of bereavement. When a family member has an emotional need to be involved in the direct care of the patient, teaching and support are provided. When a family member needs simply to talk, the staff members become the listeners.

The nursing staff also experiences its own grief process. Nurses feel the loss when a patient dies. We provide a supportive environment to help the staff deal with the emotional intensity of working with dying patients and families suffering loss. Respect and sensitivity for each other are equally as important as our sensitivity to the patients and their families.

Nursing is enhanced by close work with an interdisciplinary team and shared inservice education with others throughout the hospital. Collaboration occurs at Calvary, and we appreciate the fact that a team philosophy is at work. The interprofessional approach is valued and encouraged while never losing sight of the nurse's special role.

Education and development of staff members in all roles are major objectives. Educational opportunities are offered not only to our staff, but to visiting students as well. We welcome opportunities to teach local communities and other health institutions. Within this educational milieu, nursing research is encouraged in areas where the quality of care may be improved. A prime example of this was the development of the Cancer Care Technician Program.

Cancer Care Technician Program

In 1962, the Dominican Sisters of the Sick Poor introduced an alternative model for delivery of patient care. Determined to continue the Calvary philosophy of promoting quality care for this patient population, the Sisters developed the Cancer Care Technician (CCT) Program.

Nursing standards of care provide guidelines for the most frequently used nursing diagnoses, e.g., impaired skin integrity, malnutrition, impaired coping mechanism, increased risk for safety, bleeding precautions, and infection. Most patients require frequent turning and skin care, feeding assistance by mouth or tube, dressing changes every shift, frequent oral or tracheal suctioning, ostomy and fistula care. Isolation, hemorrhage, seizure and safety precautions are common and given the debilitated state of these patients require frequent hands-on care in order to assure comfort and dignity. The nurse and CCT work as a team to meet the patient's ongoing needs.

In the hours of anguish, fear, and loneliness that face every cancer patient, a CCT provides relief of suffering by helping both the patient and family. The use of CCTs affords the nurse additional time for the duties that can be performed only by a professional nurse. The nurse manages the specific aspects of the care of a patient and is responsible for achieving specific outcomes. The nurse can delegate components of care to a patient care assistant and supervises this care to ensure that the appropriate action has been taken.

Overview of the Program

The CCT Program, under the direction of the professional nursing staff, still affords Calvary an effective model for the delivery of quality patient care. The model is based on the premise that the professional nurse and CCT roles are highly esteemed and that they have respect for each other as caregivers.

The CCT Program is managed by the professional nurse although Calvary's modified version of Primary Nursing for patient care delivery places the technician in a key role to provide care. A procedures checklist illustrates which tasks are assigned to the technician.

Equal participation, good communication and collaboration are key components of an effective program. It leads to the development of successful team work and can achieve quality care and job satisfaction at all skill levels.

The use of patient care delivery models that include Unlicensed Assistive Personnel (UAPs) such as Calvary CCTs is increasing in acute care hospitals. With these changes occurring in skill mix, nurses are moving from responsibility for delegating certain patient care tasks, while retaining accountability for achieving nurse-defined outcomes. The nurse develops the nursing care plan, and then selects activities that may be delegated to UAPs. This manner of providing care is presumed to lower the cost of care per day and to increase nursing productivity.[1]

Under the supervision of the professional nursing staff, the CCT performs technical procedures such as stoma care, enteral feedings, complex dressing care, turning, and oral suctioning. These are performed by the technicians as delegated by the nurse. The nurse functions as care manager and overseer. This permits the time to communicate with families and other professionals, another essential and critical element of quality care. Prerequisite to this CCT and nurse relationship is training.

Training and Education

The criteria for admission to the CCT Program begins with self or peer nomination. After one year of employment, the training program affords the Nurse's Aide the opportunity to advance within the Nursing Department as a CCT.

The core class requirement of the CCT Program includes the study of physiological, psychosocial, environmental, and spiritual needs of the patient for which the CCT must demonstrate applied competence. In addition to learning physical care regimens and body systems, communication skills are an integral part of the curriculum. These include but are not limited to working well with others, sound judgment, initiative, organizational skills, dependability, quality and quantity of work, excellent communication, good appearance, courtesy, and sensitivity.

Upon completion of the six month training program, Calvary's CCT will have mastered the following:

Increased understanding of the nature of the terminally ill cancer patient;

Anatomy and physiology of adult and geriatric patients;

Description of common alterations in structure and function as a result of cancer and treatment;

Physiological, environmental, safety, spiritual, cultural, and psychosocial needs of the patient and family;

Observation skills necessary to identify altered patient physiology;

Common patient and family emotional responses to an incurable diagnosis;

Fundamental nursing care skills and theory.

There are four levels for a paraprofessional at Calvary: Nurse's Aide, Cancer Care Technician I (CCT I), Cancer Care Technician II (CCT II Instructor) and Cancer Care Technician III (CCT III Instructor Supervisor.) Here, the CCT is given the opportunity to pursue a formal course of professional nursing education through onsite college programs and a liberal tuition refund program. This program also proves advantageous for the Hospital as well as the staff because the end result is a nursing professional who knows, understands and is committed to the philosophy and spirit of Calvary Hospital.

The CCT complements the multidisciplinary approach to advanced cancer care at Calvary. Most of these patients are nutritionally at risk and the CCT has a key role in the delivery of nutritional care. They are a valuable resource for the dietitian since their hands-on care places them at the bedside. Their responsibilities include assisting the patients with daily menu completion, providing nourishments and between-meal feedings. The interaction between the dietitian and technician allows for further refinement of the patient's nutritional care plan for improved satisfaction and tolerance.

In addition to the required didactic syllabus, the CCT must demonstrate competency in the performance of many technical skills and demonstrate an increased understanding of the nature of advanced cancer in relationship to all body systems.

To assure ongoing training, the CCT is assigned to a unit under supervision of a Nurse Manager (Registered Nurse) and a Cancer Care Technician Instructor (paraprofessional) as preceptor. This team approach is fundamental to the success of the program and effective care.

Providing high quality, efficient care can be accomplished if the following conditions prevail:

Recognition of the contribution that a technician can make;

Determination of the skill level needed and assurance that the characteristics of the worker are carefully considered;

Competency-based education is initiated at the start of the change and continued to assure competency long term;

Evaluation systems are in place to assure appropriate patient outcomes and skill level competency of all staff;

Feedback and rewards are built in for all team members and teamwork is encouraged and supported;

Patient care is planned and supervised under the RN's direction so that care is RN directed, not RN intensive;

Skill mix and adjustment are based not just on allocating tasks but also on identifying how those tasks relate to the patient's severity of illness.

The CCT program has been used as a model for many other hospitals. Issues surrounding costs have compelled nurse executives to restructure nurses' work. Therefore, a restructured skill mix is central to the success of redesigned patient focused models of nursing care. Many leaders are creating staffing models that include technicians, and/or a paraprofessional that may also be called a Patient Care Assistant (PCA.) Registered nurses may delegate non-nursing tasks and responsibilities to these PCAs. Calvary sponsors a Train-The-Trainer Program for educators of other hospitals that wish to develop a technician program.

Clearly, there is much room for nursing research on the cost and quality of a care delivery model utilizing UAPs. Professional Nursing Committees should be empowered to take the initiative in this effort. The CCT Program is highly recommended to any Nursing Department seeking innovative ways to change skill mix.

Above all, we care about our patients enough to make a difference - an essential difference.

Reference

1. Spitzer-Lehmann and Roxanne. Nursing Management Desk Reference -- Concepts, Skills, and Strategies. Philadelphia: W.B. Saunders, 1994.

Portions of this paper were excerpted from the sections on Philosophy and Theory of the Calvary Nursing Manual.

ENTEROSTOMAL THERAPY SERVICES
Catherine Kalinski and Mary Schnepf

The Enterostomal Therapy services at Calvary Hospital are provided by a team of two certified Enterostomal Therapists (E.T.). They are members of the Wound, Ostomy and Continence Nurses Society (WOCN), a national association of E.T. nurses who deliver expert care to individuals with wounds, pressure ulcers, fistulae, ostomies, and incontinence. The E.T. team provides direct care on a referral basis by the physician, nurse, and/or Cancer Care Technician (CCT) to inpatients, clinic and home care patients. In addition, the E.T. provides extensive education and guidelines to staff, patients, and family members.

Due to large draining tumors, wound dehiscence, fistulae, pressure ulcers and ostomies odor is a common and challenging problem at Calvary Hospital. The interventions described have proven effective in reducing odor associated with these problems.

Essential to any odor control program is skin and wound cleanliness. In addition to frequent cleaning with Ph balanced soap and water, Desitin and Carrington moisture barriers have been found to be the products of choice for protecting the skin integrity of incontinent patients. For patients with recto-vaginal fistulae, Uni-Wash and Carrington cleansing foam are soothing, effective cleansing and deodorizing agents.

While basic skin care is very important, some solutions may be necessary prior to dressing changes and can be employed on a trial and error basis for each individual patient.

Normal Saline (0.9%) is always appropriate as a physiologic solution that flushes off surface debris but does not exert a chemical action.

Acetic Acid (0.25%) acts against gram negative and gram positive organisms, including Pseudomonas.

Hydrogen Peroxide (0.75% - 3%) effervesces and aids in removing necrotic tissue, bacteria and other debris from wound surfaces. It should not be used on new epithelium. It should only be used on open areas from which oxygen bubbles can escape.

Dakins (0.5% Sodium Hypochlorite) releases chlorine which has a bacteriocidal effect and is especially effective in wounds with malodorous drainage. This solution should only be used on a short term basis because it interferes with coagulation.

Iodophor (Povidone Iodine) acts against spores, viruses, fungi, and bacteria (including staphylococcus and anaerobes). It must be used judiciously as it may be absorbed and lead to elevation of serum iodide levels. Patients may also develop sensitivities to the iodine.

Cara-Klenz is formulated with a wetting agent and blend of moisturizers. It softens eschar and assists in removal of particulate matter without harm to living tissue. Cara-Klenz is pH adjusted for compatibility with the wound so as to aid rapid healing. Flushing with this solution can also prepare the wound for application of a dressing.

Odor associated with wounds may be effectively reduced through frequent, appropriate dressing changes. Ointments often used in wound preparation include Triple Antibiotic Ointment, Chloresium ointment, Carrington Gel and Intra Site Gel.

Exu-dry, Hydrosorb and Sorbsan are dressings which may be effectively used for heavily draining wounds. Another way to help control odor from draining fistulae, wounds and tumors is to pouch the area. There are many odor proof pouches on the market and some may be adapted so as to control heavy drainage. The Wound Manager from Squibb-Convatec has been found to be especially effective as it contributes to patient comfort and cleanliness by keeping the patient's skin dry and free from odor. This product can remain in place for several days thus reducing the frequency of dressing changes.

Pouching, which may promote overall patient comfort is also an effective means of controlling odor. It prevents drainage from leaking tubes, i.e., gastrostomy tubes. Pouching over the tube with a Universal Catheter Access Port enables containment of drainage while allowing access to the tube.

Other techniques which can be highly effective, include the use of the female urinary pouch and the fecal incontinence collector (Hollister). The female urinary pouch, a one piece disposable system, collects urine by encompassing the vulva. The Fecal Incontinence Collector is a one piece disposable perineal system which collects stool by containing the perineal areas.

Some simple but useful measures may serve as adjuncts to frequent dressing changes and appropriate pouch selection. Tic Tacs or a ½ teaspoon of mouthwash may be placed directly in a pouch. Two or three drops of oil of peppermint can be placed on the outside of a dressing at each dressing change. Derifil tablets, taken internally may be effective for some patients.

Environmental odor control products that have been found to be effective include:

3-5 drops of oil of peppermint placed in water under the bed;

Electric air kemp machine containing a solid air freshener;

Carrington odor eliminator spray;

Wiping furniture and overhead table with witch hazel;

Disposal of all dressings in a leak-proof bag upon removal.

The enterostomal therapy service has become an integral part of the nursing service. It has contributed immensely to the patients well being and relief of suffering.

CACHEXIA OF CANCER
James E. Cimino

Malnutrition and cancer are intrinsically connected. The occurrence of malnutrition in the patient with advanced cancer is so prevalent that an emaciated patient in this country is almost always first thought to have a malignant disease. In the evaluation of the prevalence of symptoms at the time of the initial interview of 1,592 Hospice patients, three quarters of the patients admitted to difficulties of eating, weight loss and dry mouth.[1] This was a prospective study and, therefore, the data is much more dependable than if it had been done retrospectively. In a 1980 study of over 3,000 cancer patients, the effect of weight loss on survival was overwhelming.[2] The median survival was significantly shortened in those patients who had weight loss of over 5% and this was found in almost every category of cancer including those malignancies that are not noted for being associated with weight loss. At Calvary Hospital, virtually every patient has lost weight by the time of admission and is at nutritional risk for malnutrition. Unfortunately, replenishing the weight loss will not in itself improve prognosis.

It is generally agreed that when evaluating the prognosis in cancer patients the following factors must be considered:

1. Type of tumor.
2. Stage of disease.
3. Weight loss, particularly of lean body mass.
4. Performance status.
5. And most importantly the availability of cancer therapy.

Without effective therapy, prolonged survival is unlikely.

The causes of cachexia are varied. No one cause is dominant. Anorexia interferes with the intake of nutrients and can play a pivotal role in causing cachexia. However, abnormal host intermediary metabolism is often more important. If the causes of anorexia are circumvented by aggressive tube feeding or parenteral nutrition, we may still not be able to correct these metabolic effects.

It is important to review what happens in other situations which lead to malnutrition. The expected metabolic effects of uncomplicated starvation in a normal person are: the resting energy expenditure (REE) decreases; the glucose falls and because of the significant utilization of fat, ketosis occurs. Since the body can maintain only limited carbohydrate stores in the form of glycogen, the body must then turn to protein breakdown and gluconeogenesis to supply the obligatory glucose. In order to minimize the amount of glucose needed, the body depends very heavily on fat for its energy substitute. Although it is characteristic to have protein catabolism decrease during simple starvation, this catabolism is never completely eliminated.

Following physical stress such as injury, trauma or surgery the patient demonstrates hypoglycemia then hyperglycemia due to insulin resistance; increased protein catabolism; a mild ketosis; and a reversal of the glucagon to insulin ratio of 1 to 4 to a ratio of 4 to 1. The resting energy expenditure (REE) increases markedly.

In the advanced cancer patient, some important differences occur. Insulin resistance is present resulting in glucose intolerance, delayed glucose clearance, abnormal insulin secretion, increased glucose production, increased glucose turnover, and increased gluconeogenesis. In some tumors, an increased Cori cycle activity has been demonstrated; glucose is converted into lactate in the tumor and the lactate is in turn converted back to glucose in the liver. This results in net waste of energy. How important a part this plays is difficult to measure.

Fat metabolism in these patients results in an excessive depletion of body fat. There is often an increased lipolysis, an increase in fatty acid production, and increased glycerol turnover rates. Glucose infusion fails to suppress the fatty acid oxidation that ordinarily would occur in the non-cancer bearing host. Decreased serum lipoprotein lipase activity is also present and contributes to the fat depletion by preventing efficient deposition.

Studies of protein metabolism in the cancer patient reveal that there is an increased whole body protein turnover, persistent muscle protein breakdown, reduced muscle synthesis, and an increase in liver protein synthesis. This increased hepatic protein synthesis is in contrast to that seen in simple starvation.

A review of the mechanisms mediating cancer cachexia was published in 1995 in *Cancer*.[3] All of these metabolic abnormalities can occur singly or in combination in virtually any advanced cancer patient. What is often seen in advanced cancer patients is really the result of a combination of these different physiological states: cancer, starvation, and stress all occurring at the same time.

Upon admission to Calvary Hospital, patients are classified according to two categories of nutritional care. These categories are comfort care and nutritional repletion. Patients who are not likely to benefit from supplemental nutritional support receive comfort care. These are patients who appear to have a very short prognosis of days to a few weeks of life. The primary goal in the care of these patients is comfort and patient satisfaction. Therapeutic diets play a very limited role in their care.

Patients whose prognosis is estimated to be over one month of life and are considered possible beneficiaries of more aggressive nutrition support have the potential for nutritional repletion. They will be given appropriate assessment and ongoing evaluation of weight, serum albumin, Na, lymphocyte count, and functional status. These patients may improve enough to be discharged either home or to nursing homes. If their nutritional status cannot be maintained, or if it worsens, they will at some point be reclassified as comfort care.

Simple and readily available laboratory tests can be used to help evaluate the nutritional status of our patients at the time of admission. A review of 100 consecutive patients admitted to Calvary Hospital revealed the following:

Serum albumin < 3.5gms per/dl = 95%

Serum albumin < 3.0gms per/dl = 80%

Total lymphocyte count <1500 = 78%

Total lymphocyte count < 1200 =72%

This pattern continues to be seen in our patients. These laboratory findings accompanied by weight loss indicate a severely malnourished group of patients.

Reviews of studies done to evaluate the value of aggressive nutritional support have invariably demonstrated either little effect or a negative effect on outcome. The position paper of the American College of Physicians, published in the Annals of Internal Medicine in 1989, concluded that "the evidence suggests that parenteral nutritional support (in chemotherapy patients) was associated with net harm, and no conditions could be defined in which such treatment appeared to be of benefit."[4] Although enteral nutrition may prove to be more beneficial, it remains to be proven. As early as 1956, in a very simple experiment, Terpeka and Waterhouse, via enteral feeding, aggressively fed nine advanced cancer patients.[5] Although the patients gained weight, it was primarily in the form of water and fat. The weight gain could not be sustained, but more important, at least half of the patients suffered detrimental effects. Since then, studies with more sophisticated measurements have demonstrated that even when patients gain weight with the most optimal nutritional intervention, it is unusual to be able to bring about positive nitrogen balance with improvement in lean body mass unless the *cancer is controlled*. Patients who do gain weight, gain water and fat. Nutritional support in the advanced cancer patient remains a frustrating and disheartening exercise. Although there is a better understanding of the cachectic state particularly in the role that cytokines may play, we do not yet know how to attack these metabolic abnormalities.

Many therapeutic interventions have been tried - modification of diet, hydrazine, anabolic hormones, insulin, cyproheptadine, cytokine antagonists, cannabinoids, immunomodulators, indomethacin, and megesterol. Only megesterol can be recommended as a practical intervention at this time and even megesterol has only limited value. An excellent review of the pharmacological options for the treatment of cachexia was published in June 1997 in *Nutrition in Clinical Practice*.[6]

Then what to do? Until we better understand this complex process, we should do the best we can, but certainly not aggressive intervention in the advanced cancer patient with a metabolically active tumor that can not be treated. Use caution when replenishing malnourished patients. The "Refeeding Syndrome" must be avoided. Go slowly and follow weights, edema, blood pressure, dyspnea, electrolytes, blood sugar, phosphorous, and potassium. The patient should be carefully evaluated for a set period, i.e., two weeks, and if not benefited, the aggressive approach should be discontinued. In our patients, nourishment is often more important psychologically then it is physiologically and food is more than nutrition.

References

1. Reuben DB, Mor V, Hiris J. Clinical symptoms and length of survival in patients with terminal cancer. Arch of Inter Med 1988; 148: 1586-91.

2. DeWys WD, Begg C, Lavin PT, et al. Prognostic effect of weight loss prior to chemotherapy in cancer patient. Am J Med 1980; 69: 491-7.

3. Toomey D, Redmond HP, Bouchier-Hayes D. Mechanisms mediating cancer cachexia. Cancer 1995; 76: 2418-26.

4. American College of Physicians: Parenteral nutrition in patients receiving cancer chemotherapy. Ann Intern Med 1989; 110: 734-35.

5. Terpeka AR, Waterhouse C. Metabolic observations during the forced feeding of patients with cancer. Am J Med 1956; 20: 225-38.

6. Herrington AM, Herrington JD, Church CA. Pharmacologic options for the treatment of cachexia. Nutr Clin Pract June 1997; 12: 3, 101-13.

CALVARY HOSPITAL'S NURTURING TRADITION
Elizabeth D. Looney

Nutrition, eating, food, and nutrients are all terms that are synonymous with nurturing. While food is that which is used to nourish the body, it can also serve many other nonphysiologic functions.

Food is often used as a symbol to represent something intangible, something that cannot in and of itself be represented, expressed or visualized. An example is the offering of food to new neighbors as a welcoming gesture to promote friendship. Food serves as a visible offering of sympathy to a grief-stricken family at a time of serious illness or the death of one of its members. The warmth and security of family and ties to home have deep associations with food. Food has the capacity to express sentiments of friendship, affection, comfort, and security. It plays an important role in satisfying not only physical needs but social, emotional and psychological needs as well. Thus the symbolism of food becomes even more significant at a time of illness, especially terminal illness.

Years of service to our patient population have provided the framework and setting for the development of the "Non-abandonment philosophy of patient care" (i.e., care that goes beyond the usual standards of accepted basic care to avoid negligence).[1] The Nutritional Care Program is a practical application of the non-abandonment philosophy and is designed to meet the unique and specific needs of patients with advanced cancer. It relies on the commitment of knowledgeable and caring professional clinical staff who see their role as significant and affecting their patients' quality of life. In addition to the Nutritional Services production and service staff, the clinical dietitians are assisted by members of the Nursing Services Department, especially nurses' aides and cancer care technicians. The nutrition-related responsibilities of these paraprofessionals include assisting the patients each morning with menu selections for the day, delivering trays, providing feeding assistance at mealtime, and delivering nourishments and between-meal feedings. These nursing staff members provide the hands-on not only of nutrition care but also other aspects of care required by advanced cancer.

Each component of the Nutritional Care Program is designed to alleviate the symptoms so frequently associated with and observed in patients with advanced neoplastic disease: anorexia, cachexia, apathy, and depression.[2] Although it is not always possible to reverse the results of the disease process, attempts to address symptoms through nutrition care can enhance patients' quality of life. This philosophy is succinctly expressed by a 15th century folk-saying: "To cure sometimes, to relieve often, to comfort always."[3]

The Initial Nutrition Assessment

Nutritional assessment is the first step in the provision of optimal nutrition care. The unit clinical dietitian initiates an evaluation of each patient's nutrition status immediately upon admission.

Anthropometrics (current weight and usual weight), laboratory assessment, clinical observation for specific indicators of nutrition inadequacies, and dietary evaluation are components of this initial assessment. Because each patient's tastes and dietary preferences are highly individual and directly affected by the disease and treatment,[4] special attention is focused on particular food items as described by the patient. References to specific foods prepared and served a special way and mention of particular brand or product names are carefully noted by the clinical dietitian. These data, when interpreted collectively, provide the basis for determining the required nutrition intervention and formulating an individualized nutrition care plan.

Two care plan levels have been established: Comfort Care and Nutritional Repletion. Comfort Care has as its goal patient satisfaction and includes accommodating patient preferences whenever possible, supportive visits (primarily through daily meal rounds) and monitoring maintaining/improving nutritional status through monitoring weight, albumin and lymphocyte levels, hydration status, recommending small frequent feeding in addition to monitoring patient's intake, tolerance and satisfaction. Initially, most patients receive Comfort Care. Continued monitoring of their acuity level, diagnosis and prognosis identifies patients who are candidates for Nutrition Repletion.

Besides providing the opportunity to collect essential information from both patient and family and/or caregivers, this admission assessment serves another purpose. Initially, it would seem almost inappropriate to hear patients or family members describe in minute detail specific food items or methods of food preparation. The lessons of time and experience, however, have taught the clinicians that focusing on foods provides respite for all involved from the uncertainties created by the transfer and admission process. For most patients, this will be their final hospital admission. The alert patient derives comfort from the pleasant associations recalled when describing a favorite food to the dietitian. Similarly, the family member is comforted when recalling the enjoyment experienced by the patient on being served a particular dish in healthier times. The anxious patient is calmed with the knowledge that a favorite security/comfort food or beverage will be provided whenever requested. As an example, knowing of the availability of apricot brandy on request calmed and eased one patient's adjustment to the new surroundings during the admission interview. The assurance of knowing that a specific item is available (although the apricot brandy was never mentioned or requested again) brings with it a sense of security that is most comforting to the patient.

Having as the goal of nutrition care improved intake and satisfaction, the clinical dietitian makes every effort to maintain each patient on as close to a regular diet as possible. Therefore, dietary restrictions are minimized, and modified diets, when indicated, are liberalized on an individual basis. Thus, the Calvary Hospital Sodium-Controlled Diet permits the use of salt in food preparation. Although processed salty foods such as bacon, cold cuts, sausages, sauerkraut, potato chips, bouillon, olives, and pickles are not included in this diet, individual patient requests for these foods are accommodated. The preparation and service of tasteless, non-seasoned food is counterproductive to the goal of nutrition care. The disease and treatment processes have already placed significant restrictions on the patients who should not have to endure further limitations at this time in their lives.

The Selective Menu

Individualized nutrition care is best achieved through the use of a selective menu. Although Calvary Hospital has a planned two week cycle menu, patients are encouraged to modify the menu each day to suit their own unique tastes and specific preferences. The most frequently requested menu substitutions include, but are not limited to, cold salads, sandwiches or platters containing meat, fish or eggs; fresh fruit with cottage cheese; omelets (plain or with filling); grilled sandwiches, and pasta dishes. Allowing patients to modify the selective menu usually results in improved patient satisfaction. A favorite food added to the menu not only may taste better to the patient but can also stimulate associations that in and of themselves are nurturing: happier, healthier times shared with loved ones and friends. These associations can be as nurturing for the patient as the food item itself.

The selective menu also enables the patient to have control over an important aspect of daily living: food selection. It is not just an issue of what is perceived and planned to be nutritious and, therefore, beneficial to the patient; rather, it is maximizing every opportunity for returning control and choice, enabling patients to have it their way.

Opportunities for choice provided by the selective menu are not limited to food. Wine and beer are also included as menu offerings. Although alcoholic beverages have been valued palliatives in virtually every culture since antiquity,[8] their use throughout history has been for pleasure rather than for health. The availability of wine, beer or a cocktail with meals was initiated with the intention of appetite stimulation in patients with advanced cancer. Although this specific goal was not achieved, a number of other positives were accomplished. The provision of an alcoholic beverage with meal service restores some degree of normalcy to patients' lives while providing additional calories and fluids. These beverages also serve as mild tranquilizers and as such can serve to improve intake at mealtime.

Similar objectives are achieved with the weekly Happy Hour. One evening each week, a group of volunteers take fully stocked portable bars to each patient unit and offer alcoholic or nonalcoholic liquid refreshments to the patients. A taste of wine, champagne or a favorite cocktail can make an evening more pleasurable and enjoyable.

The effects of the disease cannot be anticipated by the patient with advanced cancer. A feeling of well-being today can be followed by lethargy, weakness and pain tomorrow. This characteristic is also addressed through the selective menu process. Menus are distributed each morning for selection of preferences/choices for meal service on the same day. This enables patients to make their food selections based on how they are feeling on that day. This menu procedure necessitates that only breakfast selections, which usually vary minimally (on a day-to-day basis) be made one day in advance.

Breakfast and Appetite Stimulation

Experience and observation have indicated that breakfast is usually cancer patients' best meal (i.e., most enjoyed and anticipated). Although the reason for this remains unclear, one or more of the following factors provide a possible explanation. First, most patients' energy levels are highest early in the day. Second, before breakfast is probably the only time of the day when patients truly experience an appetite. The 12 - 14 hour time span since the evening meal of the preceding day has allowed for gastric emptying. Third, breakfast foods are nourishing (e.g., eggs are a rich source of biologic protein, and French toast with syrup is a nutrient - and calorie-dense food) and easy to ingest because extensive mastication or cutting is not required. In response to this patient characteristic, all efforts are directed toward the service of a high-quality, nutritious and appetizing breakfast. This is accomplished through the skills and expertise of dietary associates experienced in short-order cooking, who prepare breakfast to order for each patient in fully equipped cooking pantries located on each patient floor. The success of this unique program was aptly described by a patient who exclaimed on the first morning after her admission, "I tasted toast for the first time this morning!"

The breakfast program serves yet another important function. Although some strong cooking odors can have a negative effect on appetite in some cancer patients,[9] they can serve other patients in a positive way. This fact reinforces the need for individualization in the provision of nutrition care. The aromas of freshly brewed coffee and sizzling bacon emanating from the floor pantry can provide warm recollections of home and family. These feelings are in and of themselves nurturing and can serve to stimulate a patient's appetite or increase intake at this meal.

Meals and Early Satiety

Another aspect of the Nutritional Care Program includes addressing the problems of early satiety (i.e., the feeling of fullness) that patients often experience after ingesting minimal amounts of food. Because patients with advanced cancer are often overwhelmed by large portions, the provision of smaller portions of nutrient-dense foods served frequently is recommended.

To achieve high nutrient density, a commercial caloric supplement that does not affect the taste of foods is added in the preparation of juices and soup. Hearty, chunky soups are blenderized rather than strained for patients on puréed or liquid diets. Sauces, gravies and toppings are used to increase the caloric value of the food items prepared.

Social Activities and Care

The recognition of eating as a social behavior is an essential component in the care of patients with advanced cancer. As part of the daily routine, the clinical dietitian visits with patients during meal service. In addition to providing an opportunity to monitor patient tolerance and satisfaction with the current dietary regimen, this also allows for socialization. The celebration of religious and national holidays creates a natural setting for socialization and nurturing. Summer picnics with all the trimmings, which at Calvary are celebrated with family and friends on the outdoor patio, create a positive, pleasurable eating environment. Food, with its life-sustaining properties, is the central aspect of the Passover feast. Patients and their families derive nurturing and comfort from the sharing of the annual Passover Seder. Patients eating together can provide empathy and support for each other. Family members also receive support and strength from others who are experiencing similar pain and loss.

Enteral Feeding

The technologic advances in feeding equipment and the proliferation of available formulas over the past 20 years have greatly facilitated the feeding process for nutritionally compromised patients. An increasing number of patients are admitted to the hospital with feeding tubes already in place. Although this makes the delivery of nutrients easier, dietitians are reminded that tube-fed patients can be greatly deprived of the sensory, social and cultural associations and pleasures of eating.[10] These are pleasures consistent with quality of life that cannot be overlooked in the provision of nutrition care.

Although the tube-fed patient is unable to taste the formula being administered, flavored formulas allow the patient to "think chocolate or strawberry" or any other favorite flavor, thereby providing some degree of nurturing, comfort and pleasure. Occasionally tube-fed patients request limited tray service at mealtime, which consists of various liquids as tolerated. This affords the patient the opportunity to enjoy the pleasant aromas of nutrient-dense blended soup or the pleasure of fixing coffee or tea to his or her own liking, thus returning some degree of normalcy to mealtime. The magnitude of deprivation experienced by some tube-fed patients was poignantly verbalized by an alert, independent patient who wrote to the unit dietitian, "You don't understand, when I say heat (formula) I mean scalding...the only pleasure I experience is the warmth I feel in my stomach." The heated formula was delivered to the patient's bedside to be self-administered when the temperature was appropriate to achieve desired satisfaction.

The patient with advanced cancer provides a challenge for the clinical dietitian and other members of the health care team. The interventions described are designed to alleviate the depletion created by the disease and to focus on supporting both the physiologic and the psychologic needs of the patient. It requires that clinical staff be caring, sensitive and committed to the Nutritional Care Program, which is highly individualized, and that they recognize the significance of food as distinct from diet.[11] Food is more than nutrition.

References

1. Cimino JE. Palliative and hospice care in Calvary Hospital. Presented at Higashi Sapporo Hospital. Sapporo, Japan September 30, 1990.

2. Cimino JE. Feeding patients with advanced cancer. Diet Curr 1983; 10: pp 23-36.

3. Strauss MB., ed. Familiar medical quotations. Boston: Little, Brown & Co., 1968.

4. Carson JA, Gormican A. Taste acuity and food attitudes of selected patients with cancer. Am J Diet Assoc 1970;7: pp 361-65.

5. DeWys WD. Anorexia in cancer patients. Cancer Res 1977; 70(2):pp 354-58.

6. DeWys WD. Changes in taste sensation and feeding behavior in cancer patients. J Hum Nutr 1978; 32: pp 447-53.

7. DeWys WD. Nutrition care of the cancer patient. JAMA 1980;244: pp 374-76.

8. Kerr D. Alcohol and palliative care. Palliative Med 1992;6: pp 185-201.

9. Neilson SS, Theologides A, Vickers J. Influence of food odors on food aversions and preferences in patients with cancer. Am J Clin Nutr 1980;33:pp 235-61.

10. Padilla GV. Quoted in Habeeb MC. Eating, illness and identity. A study of the relationship of the meaning of eating and illness experience of hospitalized adults. Thesis. San Francisco: University of California, 1973.

11. MacCarthy-Levanthal EM. Post-radiation mouth blindness. Lancet 1959;2:pp 132-139.

This article was reprinted in its entirety and permission for reprint was given by Aspen Publishers, Inc. Looney E, Topics in Clinical Nutrition December, 1993; 9(1), pp 35-34.

NUTRITION SUPPORT AND NONABANDONMENT
James E. Cimino

Over the years, Calvary Hospital has developed a sophisticated feeding program that takes into account the patients' limitations and desires while trying not to place them at risk with inappropriate foods. The program tries to maximize every opportunity to feed the patient successfully. An important example of this was when the department of nutrition installed fully equipped kitchens on each patient floor. Morning is the time when patients with advanced cancer are most likely to have their best appetites, and preparing fresh and specially requested breakfast foods for the patients on their own units takes advantage of this phenomenon. The dietitians are very much involved in decision making and care of the patients.

Nourishment is often associated with life and hope, and food is symbolic of more than nourishment, even when nutrition support of the patient with advanced cancer is a frustrating exercise for patients and caregivers alike. The cases described here illustrate two different concepts regarding nourishment, and both demonstrate the practice of nonabandonment.

Case I

The patient was a 76 year-old man who had been treated for squamous cell carcinoma of the uvula one year before coming under our care. He had received maximum radical surgery, radiation therapy, and chemotherapy. A recurrence of the tumor was manifested by a mass in the neck on the ipsilateral side. This caused extreme pain locally and retroocularly. The patient had progressive difficulty in swallowing and had lost 70 pounds in approximately six months. The weight loss was attributed to both loss of appetite and his difficulty swallowing. There was no evidence of distant metastases. The patient's medical course was further complicated by transient cerebral vascular insufficiency resulting in left hemiparesis. The pain had been unremitting on a previous regimen of oral meperidine.

After coming under our care, the patient's pain was well controlled with oral levorphanol around the clock and occasional rescue doses as needed. Before the period of pain relief, the patient appeared to have accepted that he would die soon and felt that he should not undergo any further therapy. Once the pain was relieved, however, the patient's hunger and weight loss became his primary concerns. When options were discussed with him as to what might be done to lessen his weight loss and assuage his hunger, he chose to have a gastrostomy feeding tube placed.

This decision surprised his family and his caregivers. It had been clearly explained that this procedure would probably lead to some improvement, but would in no way treat the cancer and might eventually result in prolongation of suffering and pain. The complications of a gastrostomy feeding tube were also explained to him. This included discussion of the possibilities of leakage, aspiration, and infection at the site of tube placement. Nevertheless, the patient wished to go ahead with the procedure, and it was accomplished without incident. At about that time, he developed a lesion of the right lung. This proved to be an infectious process that cleared after a prolonged course of antibiotic therapy.

The patient gained weight during a period of two months. During the same time, however, the tumor mass appeared to grow at a more rapid rate than previously. The patient completely lost the ability to swallow. The tumor mass became necrotic, resulting in a fungating lesion that eventually communicated with the posterior pharynx. The patient developed further infection and then complete left hemiplegia. He died within a few days of that event, three months after the gastrostomy procedure. He was never abandoned during these final months.

The patient never expressed any regret about having had the gastrostomy tube placed. He was a rather stoic person who had strong religious convictions and was said to be a giving person. He did not express a fear of dying. We were not able to determine what he himself thought of his quality of life as a result of the feeding tube placement. The tube itself caused few discomforts. Late in the course of his disease he did develop gastric retention, which necessitated discontinuing the feedings for two days. Whether the feeding enhanced the growth of tumor is a matter of speculation. There have been a number of studies presenting evidence that, in certain animal models, aggressive feeding does result in enhancement of tumor growth. Torosion discussed stimulation of tumor growth by nutrition support in both animals and humans.[1] This is a decided risk. From a practical point of view, because malnutrition itself can lead to death, the risk of feeding may be justified even if tumor growth is enhanced. It is only when the feeding itself becomes a traumatic experience or a severe burden to the patient that one can expect most patients to forego feeding.

Case 2

This case illustrates a different attitude about feeding. The patient was a 76-year-old woman with carcinoma of the breast that had metastasized throughout her body, causing a significant degree of pain in her bones. The patient also had chronic obstructive lung disease. She had some diminution of appetite but was still able to eat. Weight loss was gradual and not overwhelmingly pervasive. The patient had always been a vigorous individual. She never wished to be dependent and wanted to have complete control of her life. She claimed not to fear death and inquired openly about her prognosis. She wanted to know whether there was any significant chance that she could be physically active again.

Because it was inevitable that her course would be one of deterioration, we had to point out to her that it was not reasonable to think that her disease would abate. It was unlikely that she could ever be fully ambulatory and independent. Her pain appeared to be well controlled with narcotics. Within a few days, the patient made the decision that she would no longer eat. She would prefer to have her dying process hastened rather than prolonged. She was quite adamant. She had discussed this decision with all her family members, who understood her well and wished to support her in any way they could. The patient appeared to have the capacity to understand the situation and was not experiencing what could be categorized as a classic depression although a trial of antidepressant therapy was given. She and her family were interviewed by the nursing staff, social worker, attending physician, psychiatrist, and dietitian. It was not possible for her to be at home because she still required medical support. We felt that we should give her the comfort that she required and be prepared to offer her nutrition, if she should have a change of mind.

The patient's deterioration was slow during the next two weeks, and she herself was questioning why she was not feeling much weaker than she did. We noted that, although the patient had continued fluids, her main fluid intake consisted of a carbonated drink of approximately 13 calories per ounce. It probably contributed 400 calories of nutrition support per day. We debated whether it was our obligation to inform her of the caloric intake from her liquids. The situation was resolved by her either recognizing this herself or being informed by other confidants. Nevertheless, once the patient became aware of the caloric intake from her beverage, she insisted that she be given only diet soda. Within one week of that episode, the patient developed an overwhelming pulmonary infection and died.

This patient made a definite choice about managing the last stage of her life, much as she had done throughout her lifetime. There was a good deal of concern, however, over whether we or others had contributed to her decision. Everyone involved made a sincere effort to make the patient understand the consequences of her action, and were prepared to stand by her in any way necessary. The dietitian gave constant support and understanding and visited her daily. This patient never asked that we assist her in actively hastening her death. When one considers the caregivers' alternatives of either discharging her to a situation where she could not get the same support for her other symptoms or literally force feeding her, the choice was obvious. Those involved in her care felt that what was done for her was the best that could have been done under the circumstances. She was not abandoned at any time.

Nutrition Support Strategies

In spite of the successes of hospice programs and the public's readiness to discuss limitations of curative care of the patient with advanced cancer, we are witnessing an increase in aggressive nutrition support for many of these patients. The newer technologies for gastrointestinal feeding tubes and vascular devices are readily available, making it easier to administer fluid and nutrients. Once started, there is a reluctance to stop either feeding or intravenous fluids, even when they are not helpful. If the treatment is inappropriate, there should be no medical, ethical, or moral distinctions between withholding and withdrawing of treatment.[2] When nourishment is equated with life and hope, it can be particularly frustrating for the caregiver not to be able to nourish the patient. If we do subject the patient to procedures or regimens that are either uncomfortable or potentially hazardous, then we certainly must have some degree of confidence that these will prove to be effective in meeting the patient's goals. This is in keeping with the standards for good medical care. Most patients who have advanced cancer undergo a number of abnormal physiological changes. What we observe in the patient is the net result of these different physiologic conditions occurring at the same time.[3,4] The changes due to inadequate nourishment are only part of the patient's deterioration.

As early as 1956, in a simple experiment, Terpeka and Waterhouse[5] aggressively fed nine patients with advanced cancer. Although the patients gained weight, it was primarily in water and fat. The weight gain could not be sustained, but even more importantly at least half the patients experienced detrimental effects. Since then, studies with more sophisticated measurements have demonstrated that, even when patients gain weight with the most optimal nutrition intervention, it is unusual to be able to bring about positive nitrogen balance and therefore unusual to improve lean body mass, except when the cancer itself is brought under control. Reviews of studies to evaluate the value of aggressive nutrition support have invariably demonstrated either little effect or negative effect on outcome.[6,7] The position paper of the American College of Physicians published in 1989[8] concluded that parenteral nutrition support in chemotherapy patients appears to be associated with net harm and that no conditions can be defined in which such treatment appears to be of benefit.[8]

Nutrition support in the patient with advanced cancer remains a difficult task. We do not know how to attack the metabolic abnormalities in most of these patients. Of all the pharmacologic interventions that have been tried, including hydrazine, anabolic hormones, insulin, cyproheptadine, cytokines, and immunomodulators, only megestrol appears to offer some possible benefit to selected patients.[9]

Ethical Decision Making

The ethics and morality involved in the management of both these patients are certainly subjects for discussion and debate. Feeding is considered, by many ethicists in our culture, a minimal means and therefore obligatory in support of the patient.[10,11] Because the kinds of nutrition support that we are presently utilizing may not benefit these patients and may even increase their suffering, it does not seem reasonable that feeding should always be considered a minimal means. There is general consensus that futile therapy should not be used, but the debate on the definition of futility continues.[12] If we define futility in terms of not being able to extend significantly a comfortable life, it would appear on the surface that the nature of the nutrition support for either of these patients could have been considered futile or inappropriate. Yet if we evaluate it in terms of what each patient perceived as an appropriate choice, then in neither situation should their respective choices be considered futile. Both patients appeared to have made autonomous and reasonably informed decisions. Certainly beneficence and autonomy were the motives of the caregivers. Their actions can even be extended to incorporate the concept of the ethics of caring[13] or, to paraphrase, the ethics of nonabandonment. This incorporates what might be considered the universally accepted virtuous concepts of ethics, beneficence, nonmaleficence, autonomy, and justice. Both patients were supported with compassion and consideration. The care givers and family members intuitively felt that they were all doing the correct thing without necessarily defining their actions in classic ethical terminology. Others have recognized this. For example, Brewin questions the need to deliberate these issues on a philosophical basis and points out that the most caring physician may be totally ignorant of academic ethics.[14] In the case of the second patient, some of the staff felt uncomfortable over the possibility that they might, in some way, be contributing to the patient's demise. Yet they offered no alternative. None of us doubted that our support for the patient at that time in his life was appropriate.

References

1. Torosion MH. Stimulation of tumor growth by nutrition support. J Parenter Enter Nutr 1992; 16 (suppl):pp 72-75.

2. President's Commission for the Study of Ethical Problems in Medicine and Biomedical Behavioral Research. Deciding to forego life-sustaining treatment; ethical, medical and legal issues and treatment decisions. Washington, DC:US Government Printing Office; 1983.

3. Kern KA, Norton JA. Cancer cachexia. J Parenter Enter Nutr 1988; 12:pp 286-298.

4. Langstein HN, Norton JA. Mechanisms of cancer cachexia. Hematol Oncol Clin North Am 1991;5: pp 103-123.

5. Terpeka AR, Waterhouse C. Metabolic observations during the forced feeding of patients with cancer. Am J Med 1956;20: pp 225-238.

6. Koretz RL, Parenteral nutrition: is it oncologically logical? J Clin Oncol 1984; 2: pp 534-538.

7. Lipman TO. Clinical trials of nutritional support in cancer:parenteral and enteral therapy. Hematol Oncol Clin North Am 1991; 5: pp 91-102.

8. American College of Physicians. Parenteral nutrition in patients receiving cancer chemotherapy. Ann Intern Med 1989; 110:pp 734-735.

9. Tchekmedyian NS, Halpert C, Ashley J, Heber D. Nutrition in advanced cancer: anorexia as an outcome variable and target of therapy. J. Parenter Enter Nutr 1992; 16 (suppl):pp 88-92.

10. Smith WB. Judeo-Christian teaching on euthanasia. NY Med Q 1986; 6:182-184.

11. Rosner F. Withholding and/or withdrawing fluids and nutrition: an opposing view. Cancer Invest 1993; 11: pp 335-357.

12. Loewy EH, Carlson RA. Futility and its wider implications. Arch Intern Med 1993; 153: pp 429-431.

13. Noddings N. Caring: A feminine approach to ethics and moral education. Berkeley: University of California Press, 1984.

14. Brewin TB. How much ethics is needed to make a good doctor? Lancet 1993; 341:pp 161-163.

Both patient case reports were changed to avoid positive identification. This article was adapted almost in its entirety and permission for reprint was given by Aspen Publishers, Inc. Cimino JE, Nutrition support and nonabandonment. Topics in Clinical Nutrition, Vol. 9, No. 1, December, 1993, pp 29-34.

PHARMACEUTICAL SERVICES AND CONCENTRATED MORPHINE
John Grom

Pharmaceutical Services has assumed an advisory role as well as an educational role in advancing rational, patient-oriented drug therapy. The department's advisory role is embodied in its collaboration in the formulation of policies regarding the evaluation, selection and therapeutic use of medications.

The primary pharmacist concept is used at Calvary Hospital. The pharmacist is assigned a specific patient care area which allows for close monitoring of each individual patient. This helps to build closer patient-pharmacist relationships while assuring high quality pharmaceutical care. The primary pharmacist monitors the patient's drug therapy from the time of admission and throughout hospitalization. The pharmacist and nurse provide education and counseling to patients and families both at the time of discharge and during outpatient visits thus assuring that they understand their prescribed medications and the importance of compliance.

Pharmacists work closely with physicians, nurses, dietitians and other hospital staff to develop performance improvement activities which foster safe and effective drug therapy. The Pharmacy and Nutritional Services Departments have developed a Drug-Nutrient Interaction Program which has proven to be an excellent mechanism to identify, monitor and prevent clinically significant drug-nutrient interactions.

The pharmacy maintains computerized patient profiles and continuously monitors the patient's drug therapy. All medication orders are reviewed and evaluated including pertinent patient demographic information (i.e., age, sex, height, weight), past drug/medical history, allergies, drug interactions, therapeutic duplication and adverse drug reactions. When a medication order needs clarification, the pharmacist consults the physician and makes appropriate recommendations. This activity is documented as part of the Pharmacist Intervention Program and is very effective in identifying areas requiring improvement.

The Pharmacy plays an active role in the Pain Management Program at Calvary Hospital. One of its most important functions is the compounding of high concentration (50mg/ml) morphine sulfate injection to meet the specific needs of our patients.

Concentrated Morphine

Since 1977, Calvary Hospital has been compounding a high-potency morphine sulfate injection that allows for single site, high dose, intermittent injection of morphine. As specialists in the treatment of severe cancer pain, Calvary staff's experience with this preparation is extensive. It is a stable and versatile solution that has been administered i.m., s.c., i.v., and epidurally to hospitalized patients without any known complications. This pharmacy compounded, preservative free, product is not commercially available and represents a highly cost efficient, patient sensitive method of delivering high dose parenteral morphine. By using a 50mg/ml potency, 95% of our patients receive parenteral volumes of less than 2ml per injection, requiring only one injection site per dose. Because of its high potency, versatility, relative stability, lack of pain on injection, and decreased dosage volumes, we use this preservative-free preparation whenever high-dose parenteral morphine therapy is required.

Historical Perspective

The pharmacy department and the medical staff collaborated to develop a formulation of a parenteral morphine solution more potent than the 15mg/ml available at that time. The medical staff solicited the pharmacy's expertise in developing a formulation of morphine that would allow the injection of smaller volumes of fluid relative to the dose prescribed and at the same time eliminate the need for multiple injection sites and the associated pain when doses greater than 30mg were prescribed.

The pharmacy developed a sterile, non-pyrogenic morphine solution with adequate stability to allow time for appropriate quality control testing prior to use. Fifty (50) milligrams per milliliter was selected as the standard. At this potency, dose calculations of volume per dose were simplified. In addition, doses under 50mg could be administered using a syringe with an ultra fine (29 gauge) needle resulting in a virtually pain-free injection.

A general outline of our current compounding process can be found in The American Journal of Health-System Pharmacists.[1] The two-phase compounding process consists of dissolution and subsequent sterilization and packaging.

Calvary Hospital's approach to pain management, using high potency preservative free, pharmacy compounded parenteral morphine as its core, addresses many of the challenges which present in treating advanced cancer pain.

Intermittent subcutaneous morphine, when dosed appropriately, is highly effective in relieving even the most severe pain. Initial doses provide rapid relief. The patient experiences minimal discomfort on injection. Subcutaneous morphine injection eliminates the need for cumbersome IV and PCA pumps which can often act as barriers to patient-family contact during this terminal stage of life. In addition, subcutaneous injections place no limitations on a patient's mobility.

Morphine is very effective, predictable in most cases, and easily titrated to patient symptom control. The preservative-free nature of our formulation permits high dose administration via infusion, where necessary, without concern for adverse reaction to preservatives routinely found in commercially available products. In addition, the morphine formulation is extremely versatile in that it can be used to administer the effective doses seen at Calvary that range from 5 milligrams to 22 grams (22,000 milligrams) per day.

Dosing can be highly individualized, based on symptomatology. This morphine preparation offers great latitude in dosing in that nurses may administer 5 to 100mg comfortably per injection site. Each injection offers an opportunity for the nurse to interact and assess the patient. The use of intermittent injection increases patient contact when compared to patients on infusions and/or PCA pumps. When these patients are very near the end of life, personal contacts are extremely important.

Regarding pharmacy/hospital administration, morphine has demonstrated itself to be extremely cost effective at a compounding cost of 2 cents per milligram. In addition, the pharmacy may use the same formulation to prepare infusions, epidurals, and high concentration oral products. In one instance, a patient's hydromorphone dose was extremely high at more than 3 grams per day. The cost of this patient's hydromorphone infusion for one 4 month length of stay exceeded the entire annual expenditure for high potency morphine for all patients. This patient's pain management needs could have been met for a fraction of the cost using high potency, preservative free morphine infusion.

This formulation is prepared solely to meet the specific in-house needs of hospitalized advanced cancer patients. The minimum amount necessary to meet short term patient needs is compounded and allows time for quality assurance testing. This product is never sold nor redistributed.

References

1. Grom JA, Bander LC. Compounding of preservative-free high-concentration morphine sulfate injection. Am J Health-Syst Pharm 1995; 52 : 2125-27.

DRUG MONOGRAPHS
Compiled by Barbara Romeo

Drug monographs concerning commonly used medications at Calvary Hospital.

I. LAXATIVES: (See Table I)
Table I lists the most commonly used treatment options for constipation at Calvary Hospital.

II. OPIOID AGONISTS:

Individualization of therapy is the foundation of pain management. Schedule doses on an "around-the-clock" basis to help prevent recurrence of pain with an "as needed" dosing schedule, to combat break through pain. **(See Table II)** The WHO ladder begins the treatment regimen:

Step 1: For mild to moderate pain: use Aspirin, Acetaminophen, or Non-Steroidal Anti-Inflammatory drug. (unless contraindicated)

Step 2: When pain persists or increases, add an opioid. (i.e. "weak" opioids such as Codeine)

Step 3: If pain continues or becomes moderate or severe, increase the opioid potency or dose. (i.e. "strong" opioids such as Morphine, Hydromorphone)

III. ANTI-EMETICS:

The following regimens are first-line therapy for control of non-chemotherapeutic-induced nausea and vomiting at Calvary Hospital:

Metoclopramide (Reglan®):
Usual adult dosage: Oral: 10mg before meals and at bedtime
                     IM: 10mg 3 or 4 times daily and q 4h as needed

Prochlorperazine (Compazine®):
Usual adult dosage: Oral: 5-10mg 3 or 4 times daily
                     Rectal 25mg twice daily
                     IM: 5-10mg q 3-4 hours as needed (do not exceed 40mg/day)

Promethazine (Phenergan®):
Usual adult dosage: IM, Oral: 12.5-25mg q 4 to 6h as needed

Trimethobenzamide (Tigan®):
Usual adult dosage: IM, Rectal: 200mg 3-4 times daily

Rarely are the 5-HT$_3$ receptor antagonists such as Ondansetron (Zofran®) or Granisetron (Kytril®) used in our patient population. Only after the above first line therapies have failed is a trial considered.

IV. SYSTEMIC CORTICOSTEROIDS:

Utilized for their anti-inflammatory and controversial appetite stimulant properties. (See Table III)

V. BENZODIAZEPINES

Utilized for their anxiolytic and sedative/hypnotic properties. (See Table IV)

VI. HYPERCALCEMIA

The treatment of hypercalcemia of malignancy begins with hydration with or without loop diuretic therapy. Once this therapy alone fails, Pamidronate is the primarily anti-hypercalcemic agent utilized at Calvary Hospital. In addition to hypercalcemia of malignancy, Pamidronate is also approved for the treatment of Paget's Disease, osteolytic bone metastases of breast cancer and osteolytic bone lesions of multiple myeloma. The following is the recommended dosing schedule for Pamidronate for its specific indications:

Hypercalcemia of Malignancy:

Symptoms and the patient's albumin-corrected serum calcium should be considered before treatment is initiated.

To determine Albumin-corrected serum calcium (mg/dl) =
Serum calcium (mg/dl) + 0.8 (4.0 - Serum albumin (g/dl))

Moderate Hypercalcemia (corrected calcium of approximately 12-13.5mg/dl) dosage is 60-90mg. The 60mg dose is given as a single dose, intravenous infusion over at least 4 hours. The 90mg dose is infused over 24 hours.

Severe Hypercalcemia (corrected calcium of >13.5mg/dl) dosage is 90mg. The 90mg dose is given as a single intervenous infusion over 24 hours.

It is recommended that a minimum of 7 days elapse before retreatment, to allow for full response to the initial dose. The dose and manner of retreatment is identical to the initial therapy.

Paget's Disease:
   The recommended dose is 30mg in 500ml of compatible solution to be administered over 4 hours for 3 consecutive days for a total of 90mg.

Osteolytic Bone Metastases of Breast Cancer:
   The recommended dose is 90mg in 250ml of compatible solution to be administered over 2 hours every 3-4 weeks.

Osteolytic Bone Lesions of Multiple Myeloma:
   The recommended dose is 90mg in 500ml of compatible solution to be administered over 4 hours on a monthly basis.

VII. **ANTI-CONVULSANTS (See Table V)**

VIII. **ANTI-DEPRESSANTS: (See Table VI)**

IX.   **ANTIPSYCHOTIC AGENTS: (See Table VII)**

References

1. McEvoy, GK ed. AHFS 97 Drug Information. Bethesda: Society of Health Systems Pharmacists, Inc., 1997.

2. Cada, DJ. ed. Drug Facts & Comparisons 1997 with updates. St. Louis:Facts & Comparisons, 1997.

3. Aredia® Package Insert. 1997 Novartis.

TABLE I - LAXATIVES

Laxative Generic (Brand)	Class	Site of Action	Usual dosage
Bisacodyl (Dulcolax®)	Stimulant	Colon	1 suppository pr qd, 10mg po qd
Cascara Sagrada ± Milk of Magnesia	Stimulant	Colon	5ml po at bedtime
Docusate (Colace®)	Sulfactant	Small & Large Intestine	300mg po qd
Docusate & Casanthranol (Peri-Colace®)	Sulfactant/ Stimulant	Colon	1 cap po tid
Glycerin (Sani-Supp®)	Hyperosmotic	Colon	1 suppository pr qd
Lactulose (Cephulac®)	Miscellaneous	Colon	10-20g (15-30ml) po qd
Magnesium Citrate (Citroma®)	Saline	Small & Large Intestine	5-10 fl. oz. po qd prn
Magnesium Hydroxide (Phillips Milk of Magnesia®)	Saline Laxative	Small & Large Intestine	30-60ml po qd
Mineral Oil (Kondremul®)	Lubricant	Colon	30ml po qd
Psyllium (Metamucil®)	Bulk-Producing	Small & Large Intestine	1 packet po bid

TABLE I (cont.)

Senna (Senokot®)	Stimulant	Colon	2 tabs po at bedtime
Sodium Phosphate/ Biphosphate enema (Fleet®)	Saline	Small & Large Intestine	1 enema pr qd pm

TABLE II

The following table lists the approximate equianalgesic dose and usual starting dose for moderate to severe pain in adults ≥ 50 kg:

Usual Starting Dose for Opiods Drug

Opioid agonist, Generic (Brand)	Approximate Equianalgesic Dose		Moderate to Severe Pain	
	Oral	Parenteral (IM)	Oral	Parenteral (IM/SC)
Codeine	200mg	120mg	60mg q 3-4h	60mg q 2h
Hydromorphone (Dilaudid®)	7.5mg	1.5mg	6mg q 3-4h	1.5mg q 3-4h
Levorphanol (Levo-Dromoran®)	4mg	2mg	4mg q 6-8h	2mg q 6-8h
Meperidine (Demerol®)	300mg	75mg	Not Recommended	100mg q 3 h
Methadone (Dolophine®)	20mg	10mg	20mg q 6-8h	10mg q 6-8h
Morphine (MSIR®)	30mg (repeat dose) 60mg (single dose)		30mg q 3-4h	
Morphine, Calvary concentrated 50mg/ml		10mg		10mg q 3-4h
Morphine, controlled release (MS Contin®)	90mg-120mg q 12h	n/a	90-120mg q 12h	n/a
Oxycodone (Roxicodone®)	30mg	n/a	10mg q 3-4h	n/a

TABLE III - SYSTEMIC CORTICOIDS

The following is a comparative equivalency chart of the glucocorticoids commonly prescribed at Calvary:

Glucocorticoid Generic (Brand)	Approximate Equivalent Dose	Route	Relative Anti-Inflammatory Potency	Relative Mineralocorticoid Potency	Biologic Half-life
Short-Acting:					
Hydrocortisone	20mg	PO	1	2	8-12h
(Solu-Cortef®)		IM,IV	1	2	8-12h
Intermediate-Acting:					
Prednisone					
(Deltasone®)	5mg	PO	4	1	18-36h
Methylprednisolone	4mg	PO,	5	0	18-36h
(Medrol®)		IM,IV	5	0	18-36h
Long-Acting:					
Dexamethasone	0.75mg	PO,	25-30	0	36-54h
(Decadron®)		IM,IV	25-30	0	36-54h

TABLE IV - BENZODIAZEPINES

The following is a comparative chart of the commonly prescribed benzodiazepines at Calvary:

Agent Generic (Brand)	Usual Adult Oral Daily Dosage	Usual Adult IM daily dosage	Peak Oral Blood Levels	Major Active Metabolite	Half-Life (Parent)	Half-Life (Metabolite)
Alprazolam (Xanax®)	0.75-4mg	n/a	1-2h	No	12-15h	No
Diazepam (Valium®)	4-40mg	2-20mg	0.5-2h	Yes	20-80h	50-100h
Lorazepam (Ativan®)	2-6mg	0.5-4mg	1-6h	No	10-20h	No
Flurazepam (Dalmane®)	15-60mg	n/a	0.5-2h	Yes	Not significant	40-114h
Temazepam (Restoril®)	15-30mg	n/a	2-3h	No	10-40	No

TABLE V - ANTI-CONVULSANTS

Drug Generic (Brand)	Labeled Seizures Indications for	Usual Adult Daily Dosage	Therapeutic Plasma Concentration (mcg/ml)	Comments
Carbamazepine (Tegretol®)	Tonic-clonic Mixed Psychomotor	400-1200mg daily in divided doses	4-12	Aplastic anemia and agranulocytosis has been reported
Clonazepam (Klonopin®)	Absence Myoclonic Akinetic	1.5mg-20mg in divided doses	20-80	Increase in increments of 0.5 -1mg q 3 days until seizures are controlled or until side effects preclude increase
Diazepam (Valium®)	Status epilepticus Epilepsy, all forms	Oral : 2-10mg 2 to 4 times daily Parenteral: 5-10mg. Repeat q 10-15 minutes up to maximum dosage of 30mg.	not established	Parenteral therapy may be repeated in 2-4 hours, however, residual active metabolites may persist. Also indicated as an anxiolytic.
Gabapentin (Neurontin®)	Adjunctive therapy of partial seizures with or without secondary generalization	900-1800mg/day in divided doses	not established	Recommended for add-on therapy

TABLE V (cont.)

Phenobarbitol (Luminal®)	Status epilepticus Epilepsy, all forms Tonic-clonic	Oral: 60-100mg/d Parenteral: 200-320mg IM/IV repeat q 6h as needed	15-40	Also indicated for use as a sedative/hypnotic. Associated with many drug interactions
Phenytoin (Dilantin®)	Tonic-clonic Psychomotor	Oral Load: 1 gram in 3 divided doses at 2h intervals then Maintenance 24h after. IV Load: 10-15mg/kg slowly then Maintenance IV/PO Maintenance: 100mg q 6 to 8h	5-20	Associated with many drug interactions.
Valproic Acid & Derivatives (Depakene®, Depakote®)	Absence	10-15mg/kg/day in divided doses; increase by 5-4 10mg/kg/day at weekly intervals till therapeutic levels are achieved. Maintenance 30-60mg/kg/day in divided doses	50-150	Hepatic failure had resulted in fatalities in patients receiving valproic acid and its derivatives. Perform liver function tests prior to and during therapy.

TABLE VI - ANTI-DEPRESSANTS

Drug Generic (Brand)	Ususal Dosage (mg/day)	Anti-Cholinergic	Sedation	Orthostatic Hypotension	Nor-Epinephrine	Serotonin
Amitriptyline (Elavil®)	50-300	Very High	Very High	Moderate	Moderate	Very High
Desipramine (Norpramin®)	25-300	Slight	Slight	Slight	Very High	Moderate
Doxepin (Sinequan®)	25-300	Moderate	High	Moderate	Slight	Moderate
Nortriptyline (Pamelor®)	30-100	Moderate	Moderate	Slight	Moderate	High
Fluoxetine (Prozac®)	20-80	Slight	Slight	Slight	Slight	Highest
Paroxetine (Paxil®)	10-50	None	Slight	None	Slight	Highest
Sertraline (Zoloft®)	50-200	None	Slight	None	Slight	Highest

TABLE VII - ANTIPSYCHOTIC AGENTS

Drug Generic (Brand)	Approx. Equivalent dosage (mg)	Daily Adult Dosage (mg)	Sedation	Extra-pyramidal Symptoms	Anticholinergic Effects	Orthostatic Hypotension	Therapeutic Plasma Concentration (mg/ml)
Chlorpromazine (Thorazine®)	100	30-800	High	Moderate	Moderate	High	30-500
Haloperidol (Haldol®)	2	1-15	Low	High	Low	Low	5-20
Prochlorperazine (Compazine®)	15	15-150	Moderate	High	Low	Low	
Thioridazine (Mellaril®)	100	150-800	High	Low	High	High	
Trifluoperazine (Stelazine®)	5	2-40	Low	High	Low	Low	

DRUG AND FOOD INTERACTIONS
Rick Tota

Drug-nutrient interactions are defined as events and outcomes that result from physical, chemical, physiologic or pathophysiologic relationships between drugs and nutrients. They can be categorized as either diet or nutrient effects on drug therapy and drug effects on nutritional status.

The interaction or its outcome is clinically important when the therapeutic response to a drug is reduced, when it causes acute or chronic toxicity or if it can result in impaired nutritional status.

Those patients at greatest risk are:

The elderly who take more medications than any other age group

Patients with chronic diseases requiring long term use of medications

Patients with multiple drugs

Patients with poor diets.

Foods may affect the pharmacokinetics of a drug (absorption, distribution, metabolism and excretion) by altering gastric pH, secretion and gastrointestinal motility and transit time. Certain constituents in foods may chelate or adsorb the drug, resulting in a decrease in the extent and rate of its absorption. Foods may interact with drugs by influencing their effects or pharmacologic actions such as diets high in vitamin K which decrease the effects of Warfarin, or alcoholic beverages which increase the CNS depressant effects of benzodiazapines, antihistamines and opiates.

Drugs can affect nutritional status by:

Decreasing taste perception (i.e., Azathioprine, Baclofen, Carbamezapine)

Altering taste perception (i.e. Allopurinol, Captopril, Carbamezapine)

Stimulating appetite   (i.e., Antihistamines, Benzodiazepines, Hypoglycemic agents, Steroids)

Reducing appetite: (i.e. Anticonvulsants, Antineoplastics, Digitalis, Metronidazole, Thiazide, Diuretics)

Inducing nausea and vomiting (chemotherapy)

Inducing constipation (narcotics) or diarrhea (antibiotics)

Inducing vitamin and mineral deficiencies.

The majority of patients at Calvary Hospital are elderly and due to advanced cancer are frail, debilitated and malnourished. This places them at increased risk for potential drug-nutrient interactions. The Departments of Pharmaceutical Services and Nutritional Services work together to avoid potential drug-nutrient interactions. The goal is to optimize the effectiveness of drugs while maintaining proper nutritional status. They have developed a Drug-Nutrient Interaction Program which has been very effective in identifying, monitoring and preventing clinically significant interactions.

The "Drug-Nutrient Interaction Chart" provides a summary of some of the more important interactions. This chart lists the potentially interacting drugs and nutrients, the mechanism of interaction and preventive measures (see Table 1.)

References

1. Yamreudeewong W, et al. Drug-food interaction in clinical practice. Gr Fam Prac 40;(4), pp 376-384.

2. Kirk JK. Significant drug nutrient interactions, Am Fam Phys 1995; 51(5), pp 1175-1182.

3. Williams L, Davis JA, Lowenthal DT. The influence of food on the absorption and metabolism of drugs. Clin Nutr 1993; Vol 77 (4):pp 815-829.

4. Huyck N. Patient education: implementing a food and drug interactions program. Top Clin Nutr 1991; 6(3), pp 34-41.

5. Grapefruit juice interactions with drugs. Med Letter. 1995; Issue 995: 37.

6. American Hospital Formulary Service: Drug Information. 1995.

TABLE I
DRUG-NUTRIENT INTERACTION CHART

DRUG	NUTRIENT	MECHANISM	PREVENTIVE MEASURES
ACE Inhibitors: Captopril Enalapril Lisinopril	Potassium-containing salt substitutes	ACE inhibitors inhibit excretion of potassium, increase in serum potassium levels	Avoid use of potassium-containing salt substitute
Ampicillin	Regular Meal	Decreased absorption	Take on empty stomach, give 1 hr before or 2 hrs after meals
Cholestyramine	Fat soluble vitamins- A, D, E and K	Bile acid sequestrants may decrease the absorption of vitamins A, D, E, and K by interfering with activity of bile acid, an important emulsifying agent for absorption of fat soluble vitamins.	When administered for a long period of time, supplementation with water-miscible or parenteral forms of vitamin A and D may be warranted.
Ciprofloxacin	Dairy products (milk, yogurt)	Significant decrease in absorption due to complexation with divalent cations Calcium and Magnesium	Space dairy products at least two hours after Ciprofloxacin
Digoxin	Bran Fiber	Diets with high bran fiber may significantly reduce absorption of digoxin resulting in decreased serum levels	Give 1/2 to 1hr before or 4 hours after bran fiber
Erythromycin base	Regular Meal	decreased absorption	Preferably taken on an empty stomach 1hr before or 2hrs after meals, if GI upset occurs may be taken with food

DRUG	NUTRIENT	MECHANISM	PREVENTIVE MEASURES
Glucocorticoids: Hydrocortisone Prednisone	Sodium, Potassium Calcium	Can cause sodium retention, potassium loss, increase in calcium excretion	Dietary salt restriction may be advisable, potassium supplementation may be necessary
Indinavir	High caloric meal	The presence of food in the stomach can significantly decrease the absorption of Indinavir	Administer 1 hour before or 2 hours after a meal
Isoniazid	Pyridoxine (Vitamin B6), Alcohol, Vitamin D, tyramine-containing foods	Inhibits Vitamin B6, may cause hypocalcemia and hypophosphatemia due to alterations in Vit D metabolism, inhibits monoamine oxidase - can cause tyramine-like reaction	Vitamin B6 supplementation may be required, avoid daily ingestion of alcohol, avoid tyramine-containing foods
Laxatives: Milk of Magnesia	Potassium, Calcium, Magnesium	Prolonged use may decrease absorption of potassium, calcium, magnesium	
Bisacodyl	Milk	Dissolves enteric coating, may dissolve in the stomach rather than small intestine, can cause gastric irritation	Do not take with milk
Mineral Oil	Fat soluble vitamins A, D, E, and K	May result in reduced absorption of vitamin A, D, E, and K, may lead to low serum calcium and phosphate levels	

Drug & Food Interactions

DRUG	NUTRIENT	MECHANISM	PREVENTIVE MEASURES
Lithium	Low salt diet	Increase in serum Lithium levels due to increased reabsorption and possibly toxicity, can cause nausea, vomiting, diarrhea, arrhythmias, seizures	Maintain constant intake of salt and fluids to avoid changes in Lithium excretion
	High salt diet	Decrease in serum Lithium level due to increase in renal excretion of Lithium.	
Metronidazole	Alcohol	Disulfiram-like reaction- facial flushing, tachycardia or palpitations, headache, nausea and vomiting	Avoid alcohol and alcohol-containing products
Monoamine Oxidase Inhibitors: Isocarboxazid Phenylzine Tranylcypromine	Tyramine-rich foods	Increase in catecholamine levels by inhibiting their degradation, can cause hypertensive crisis	Avoid tyramine-rich foods such as: aged mature cheeses (unpasteurized-cheddar, blue, swiss), smoked or pickled meats, fish or poultry (herring, sausage, corned beef, salami, pepperoni), aged or fermented meats, fish or poultry (chicken or beef liver pate), game, yeast extract (Brewers yeast), red wines (chianti, burgundy, sherry, vermouth)
Nifedipine	Grapefruit juice	Inhibits the metabolism of Nifedipine, may increase serum concentrations	Avoid grapefruit juice

DRUG	NUTRIENT	MECHANISM	PREVENTIVE MEASURES
Phenytoin	Folic acid, Vitamin D	Phenytoin may interfere with folic acid absorption resulting in megaloblastic anemia, can also cause derangements of vitamin D metabolism resulting in osteoporosis	
	Enteral feedings	Enteral feedings can significantly reduce Phenytoin serum levels	The enteral feedings may need to be withheld 2hrs before and 2hrs after Phenytoin administration
Tetracycline	Dairy products (milk, yogurt)	Significant decrease in absorption of Tetracycline due to chelation with Calcium and Magnesium	Give 1hr before or 2hrs after dairy products
Warfarin	Vitamin K-rich foods	Vitamin K antagonizes the action of Warfarin	Maintain a balanced diet without abrupt intake of large amounts of vitamin K rich foods such as: green leafy vegetables, spinach, broccoli

SOCIAL WORK
Barbara Guilfoyle and Debbie Feldman

> The single most important thing to know about Americans is that . . . they think that death is optional.
> Jane Walmsley, *Bri-Think; Ameri-Think,* 1986

"Any serious illness afflicts families, not just individuals."[1] We know that when a person is diagnosed with cancer, the whole family "gets cancer." The struggle, however, is that very often, the family members remain the hidden victims. Family members emotional needs are often neglected by the health care system and by the community at large.

At Calvary Hospital the social worker may be the first person to ask the family, "How are you doing?" The first to understand that family emotions are directly linked to the patient's medical state. We often hear a family member say, "If my loved one is having a good day, I'm having a good day. If they are not, I'm not." Family members are so busy attempting to meet the needs of the patient and remaining/becoming informed about the patient's current condition, that they are often unaware of their own stress levels and subvert their emotional needs.

This is a time often referred to in social work literature as the period of grief. Families begin to grieve the loss of life as it was and live on a roller coaster of uncertainty. By the time a patient enters Calvary Hospital, the predominant and overriding family issue is stress. Stress in the individual and stress in the family system as a whole.

As part of the initial psychosocial assessment, a social worker is assigned to meet with the patient and the family. The worker provides palliative care services to families as well as patients during the periods of illness and anticipatory grief, as well as through the actual loss and during bereavement.

The frame work for social work intervention as practiced in a palliative care setting as contrasted in a general acute care facility is distinguished in several ways. The focus of social work interventions is on the family and the family's ability to cope. Although the patient is of primary importance, the Calvary patient tends to be too ill most of the time to attempt to do this kind of grief work. The treatment goals involve bringing family members together around the issues of death and dying. This is a crisis model where the focus is on the current issue. Social workers in this setting arrange family sessions to assess the family threshold for handling crisis, relationships in the family and the various strengths of the individual family members.

The requirements for the social worker at a palliative care hospital are unique as well. The essential requisites are that the worker must have come to understand his/her own response to death and that they must understand the process of grief as it relates to the experiences of the patient and the family. They must have exceptional listening skills and recognize personal limitations. Most importantly, as we say in social work training, a worker in this facility needs to have an understanding that you "start where the family is" and that your personal values and beliefs regarding terminal illness and death have no place in your work with this population.

Social workers, in a palliative care setting, work with two sets of tasks. These tasks are separated out in this discussion. However, in reality, it can not often be delineated so readily.

The tasks of a patient in a palliative care setting:

> Family communication patterns
> Emotional "staging"
> Making decisions regarding treatment
> Managing/participation in pain control
> Maintaining hope
> Grieving losses
> Reviewing one's life
> Taking care of unfinished business
> Taking care of day-to-day business
> Healing relationships.

It is important that as a social worker in the facility we do not make any assumptions about the level of involvement that patients want to maintain in their care. The questions need to be asked directly to the patient. How much do you want to know about what is happening? What information is helpful to you? How involved do you want your family to be in your care? The worker also assists the patient in handling any unfinished business. It is often easier for patients to articulate what they would like to say to their family with a "stranger" in the room. Many patients have used social workers in this role. The social worker rehearses the script of what the patient wants to say prior to the family meeting. The patient determines whether they want the social worker to remain in the room for assistance during the meeting. The social worker is available after the meeting for follow up with the patient and with the family. Many patients have used this opportunity to write a will of their possessions with their children or to ask for forgiveness. For example, one patient asked his adult children to forgive him for being a failure because he was an alcoholic. His children gladly forgave him and told him that they thought of him as a loving devoted father who worked two jobs to support his family and never knew that he felt this way. The patient cried and was able to die not feeling "like a failure."

The tasks of a family in a palliative care setting:

> Accepting the prognosis and dealing with their own stages of grief;
> Learning how to speak with the patient honestly but supportively;

> Coming to agreement on treatment decisions, respecting the patient's decisions;
> Caring for the dying patient;
> Adapting to changes related to the patient's illness:
> > Financial,
> > Role changes,
> > Reorganization to continue functioning;
> Meeting the needs of the dying patient.

There are several factors that may affect how a family copes with this current stressor. These include:

> What role did the patient play in the family?

From experiences we have come to know the significance of the family role. The husband of a patient spoke tearfully of the impending death of his wife, Emma. "I don't know what I'll do - I won't be able to take care of things like she did."

> How significant was this role (for example: was the person the primary bread winner?)
> What are the beliefs in the family?
> What other losses have occurred and in what time frame?

We have all come to know families where multiple losses have changed their actions, beliefs, and practices. One such family was convinced that it was "cursed" - due to its own actions - as multiple losses from cancer had occurred over a period of time. The significant education and need for preventive education is immeasurable in helping families to take actions in their own best interests.

> How intact or conflicted is the family system?
> How open or blocked is the family communication?
> How long has the patient been sick? (history of the illness and treatment).
> What additional supports exist for this family?

Families may cope with stress in very different ways. Stress may present to our staff as anxiety or it may present as anger projected outward. Anxiety and anger are often expressed when a person or a family system is out of control or when families are unable to maintain their homeostasis. It is not possible in this environment to fully understand the historical, cultural or ethnic origins of this familial stress. We are meeting families in crisis.

The treatment plan and methodology utilized is comprehensive. All of our goals are short term. We are aware that we cannot solve long-term family needs. The treatment involves a combination of psychotherapy, crisis therapy, guided imagery, and relaxation techniques. We have had an entire family in the room doing a relaxation exercise and then talking about it. For the first time in months the family was able to discuss something pleasant and share an experience that was not related to cancer, doctors, treatment, or hospital. We are looking to ensure that the patient and family can attain some level of emotional comfort around the illness and ultimate death.

Programmatically the Social Work Department offers a number of group supports as well as individual and family therapy.

> The Family Support Group meets twice a week to provide families and friends with an opportunity to express themselves in an environment of safety. Sharing common experiences with the goal of normalizing experiences is the function of the group.
>
> The Family Intervention Team (FIT) is a group of disciplines assembled ad hoc to meet with families in order to address their needs. The team is assembled when the family perceives that their needs are not being met by the interdisciplinary team and would like some additional response.

We are in the process of developing a child's support group, specifically developed to address the needs of children ages 6-12.

Another challenge in caring for patients near the end of life is knowing what the patient would like done: how aggressive is medical care to be; what are the perceptions of the burdens of treatment for the patient? In general, patients do change their minds, but those who take the time to write advance directives are less likely to change their minds. This is probably due to the fact that they did take the time and gave serious thought to their wishes.[2] The social worker plays a vital role in helping patients make their wishes known.

Since 1991 the Federal Patient's Self Determination Act mandated providing Medicare and Medicaid patients with education and the opportunity to prepare an advance directive. At Calvary Hospital it is the social worker who oversees the proper fulfillment of this requirement.

The patient may have a living will, but it is the appointment of a health care proxy that is used most frequently. It is the proxy (health care agent or surrogate) who has the authority to make health care decisions on behalf of the individual if that individual becomes incapable of making health care decisions.

If the patient does not yet have an Advanced Directive, but is able to complete one, the social worker educates the patient to his/her rights and to the value of appointing a proxy. This is done as soon after admission as is possible. It is also the right of the patient to choose not to execute a proxy.

Although almost all of Calvary patients are transferred from other health care facilities, only 20% have in place an advance directive or health care proxy. Of the remaining patients, 30% are capable of initiating a proxy on the day of admission, but only 5% (or 1.5% of all patients) choose to do so.

If a proper advance directive is lacking, the social worker will repeatedly try to have the patient complete one. A copy of the document is then placed in the medical record, along with a notation of the existence of the advance directive on the face sheet of the patient's chart.

The programs of the Social Work Services Department are constantly being evaluated and monitored to meet the needs of patients and family. Health care delivery systems are changing but the needs of patients/families continue and become even more critical in these changing times.

REFERENCES

1. Spiegel D. Living beyond limits. New hope and help for facing life-threatening illness. New York: Random House Publishers 1993; 176.

2. Davis M, Garrett J, Harris R, Patrick DL. Stability of choices about life-sustaining treatments. Ann Intern Med 1994; 120:567-73.

THERAPEUTIC RECREATION AND LIFE AFFIRMATION
Nanette Vallecillo

The fear of the unknown, the dreaded words "You have cancer; there is no more treatment to cure you" or "You are dying," replaying in a person's head. How often this scenario is repeated on a daily basis. People go through endless hours, days and months of tests, treatments and anxiety wondering is this going to help; can I dare hope? The emotional reactions and fears of a dying patient run the gamut from anxiety to rationalization. Previous hospitalizations, endless procedures and treatments have given patients and families a heightened awareness of how precious life is to them. They will often welcome life affirming interactions with others and their environment.

As part of the palliative care process the Therapeutic Recreation Service focuses on the individual patient and family by addressing quality of life issues, perceptions of their use of time in a hospital setting and control over their environment as well as creative coping strategies.

Rationale

Over the years, as therapeutic recreation was pioneered at Calvary Hospital with oncology patients who were in advanced stages of their cancer, there has been much feedback given by them on their expressed needs and concerns.

The following will be addressed throughout this article:

> The fear of suffering and pain;
> The fear of the unknown;
> The fear of increasing loss of control and independence;
> The need to feel that they will not be abandoned;
> The need to feel that they have their identity;
> The need to make choices;
> The need to feel productive;
> The need for creative expression;
> The need to feel "normal."

Therapeutic recreation interventions are used at Calvary Hospital as tools in focusing on what is important to the patient in terms of coping with their illness and increasing disabilities.

Program

Our service offers individual therapeutic recreation interventions as well as group therapeutic recreation programs on a daily basis, seven days a week. With an emphasis on proactively living, our patients enjoy using their time in a satisfying and productive manner, expressing their past lifestyle in a modified form or perhaps learning a new leisure skill.

These interventions cover a wide range of programs such as ceramics, horticulture, creative arts, crafts, relaxation/movement, games, music, special parties, as well as, individual interventions such as life review, sensory activities, reminiscing, support visits, socialization, and all of the above which can be modified on a one on one basis. The therapeutic recreation interventions, environment of care and interaction patterns are planned, structured and evaluated by qualified recreation therapists and technicians.

Therapeutic Recreation Interventions

The assessment of each patient provides the staff with the information vital to developing an individual care plan. The issue of personal control, decision making, and fear of increasing loss of independence is of great concern to patients. The predictability and order of having scheduled, structured recreation programs can be comforting to a person conferring a sense of security and anchoring. The recreation activity calendar becomes a vehicle to provide the patient and family with information to exercise personal choice and control over the use of their valuable time.

Anxiety, stress and depression will be common barriers for the patient and family. Therapeutic recreation can offer creative strategies in reducing or overcoming some difficult moments. Based on the rapport and trusting relationships developed by the Therapeutic Recreation staff during individual support visits the moment can be seized when unexpectedly a despondent patient responds to an invitation to participate in an activity, to participate in life again. It should not be presumed that, although a patient has limited expectancies about life's future, he/she does not find meaning in the present.

"Persons do things. They act, create, make, take part, put together, wind, unwind, cause to be, and cause to vanish. They know themselves, and are known, by these acts. When illness restricts the range of activity of persons, they are not themselves."[1]

So many of the patients suffer psychological or emotional pain resulting from their increasing loss of independence; increasing disabilities due to the disease process; loss of self-image and their perception of a loss of control over their environment and their choices. It is legitimate to feel stressed, anxious and depressed.

The wide range of options offered by therapeutic recreation activities can be an important tool in the palliative care process by helping the patient to relieve tension, stress, anxiety, and boredom, as well as to promote and facilitate avenues of relaxation and distraction from pain. These programs and interventions also provide constructive outlets for emotions and afford opportunities for the development of social relationships and peer support systems. The patient luncheon on the terrace during the summer months allows patients and their loved ones an opportunity to have a "normalized" lunch together which they might have had in their back yard, at home or in a restaurant.

Our Horticulture Program provides an opportunity for the patient to accomplish a gardening task and make a meaningful contribution to the patient hospital garden. It instills a sense of self-worth in many patients, improving their mental health at a crucial time. Even the patient with a few weeks to live gains satisfaction at viewing that plant on their window sill or the garden that will bloom year after year as a living memorial.

Creative expressions through a "writing/poetry" session during our Creative Arts Program allows a mother to tell her children whom she will not see grow up that she will be there with them through the words she leaves behind. During current event discussions, opinions and viewpoints are solicited. Learning can still happen by acquiring new leisure skills through ceramics or crafts, giving the patients a sense of accomplishment and purpose when they, for example, make a gift for a significant other, perhaps a birthday gift for their grandchild.

Promoting friendships and laughter can reduce tension. Patients and families feel more "UP" when the seriousness and sadness of cancer is dispelled by use of humor. Volunteers sometimes dress up in comical outfits or add levity to the conversation during word games or social group sessions.

"It relieves tension and anxiety, serves as an outlet for hostility and anger, and allows a temporary escape from reality." "Humor helps to break the ice, encourage trust, reduces the fear of the unfamiliar setting, and establishes positive relationships among patient, family and staff."[2]

People have a basic need to be loved, to be needed, to be wanted, to be welcomed, to still be a part of life. Everyone's daily existence includes a leisure lifestyle and how we express this lifestyle will differ with each person, but the fact remains that each person has one.

"Persons have regular behaviors. In health, we take for granted the details of our day-to-day behavior. Persons know themselves to be well as much by whether they behave as usual as by any other set of facts. Patients decide that they are ill because they cannot perform as usual, and they may suffer the loss of their routine. If they cannot do the things that they identify with the fact of their being, they are not whole."[1]

Although uprooted from their "normal lifestyle and identity" they can still take pleasure in sharing life affirming experiences. Sharing with friends, their fears, pain, suffering, hopes, and dreams, can bring comfort and foster a caring environment through which the journey may be better tolerated. To laugh and cry together is the Calvary way.

References

1. Cassell EJ. The nature of suffering and the goals of medicine. N Engl J Med 1982; No. 11 643.

2. Bellert JL. Humor: a therapeutic approach in oncology nursing. Cancer Nursing. 1982; Vol 12. No. 2 66-67.

VOLUNTEERS
Mary Ann Gulla

Volunteers have a long history in caring for the sick and particularly for those patients at the end of life. In our country it is an integral part of many of our institutions. Alexis de Tocqueville documented his experiences and observations about our political, social and cultural institutions in his book, *Democracy in America*. He went so far as to credit the very success of our democratic system to the voluntary association:

> They have not only commercial and manufacturing companies, in which all take part, but voluntary associations of a thousand other kinds, religious, moral, serious, futile, general or restricted, enormous, or diminutive. The Americans make associations to give entertainments, to found seminaries, to build inns, to construct churches, to diffuse books, to send missionaries to the antipodes; in this manner they founded hospitals, prisons, and schools.

> When an American asks for the cooperation of his fellow citizens, it is seldom refused; and I have often seen it afforded spontaneously, and with great goodwill. If an accident happens on a highway, everybody hastens to help the sufferer; if some great and sudden calamity befalls a family, the purses of a thousand strangers are at once willingly opened and numerous donations pour in to relieve their distress.[1]

The founders of the Calvary program were volunteers. It was because of just such a group called Women of Calvary, who possessed the characteristics of compassion, concern and willingness to give of themselves, that the House of Calvary began in 1899. Their spirit of commitment, concern and non-abandonment continues through the entire hospital staff and particularly in our volunteer program.

Calvary is staffed with competent professionals who really care. It has been the goal of the Volunteer Services Department to affirm this goal and to attract volunteers from the local community; people and friends who are willing to share their talents, time, compassion, and sensitivity. These special people complement our staff by adding to the quality of life for patients and by reaching out to their families. Some of the volunteers are inspired by a particular experience they may have had. Either a loved one was cared for at Calvary Hospital or they may have lived through the suffering illness of another person or heard about our work and want to help. Whatever the reason, they are all highly motivated and understand that they can make a difference.

Presently we have 200 volunteers whose donated hours translate into fourteen full time equivalent positions. Each volunteer is interviewed individually and screened for his/her capacity to relate to the environment of Calvary Hospital. Following a general orientation, the volunteer is placed in a department and given an inservice task specifically related to that department. Upon mutual agreement of both the volunteer and department head, the volunteer will then continue the assignment. The Director of Volunteers, her Assistant and fellow volunteers, are all available for consultation and support of the new volunteer.

It is very important that the volunteer not be in a state of unresolved grief, since this can be the greatest deterrent to a volunteer's successful performance.[2] We require a waiting period of one year after the death of a significant other before allowing a volunteer to work with patients. Some years ago a woman, whose husband had died of cancer at Calvary Hospital six months earlier, offered to volunteer. I suggested that she wait at least another six months but she insisted. She prevailed on us by offering a letter from her physician indicating that she was well adjusted and should be very successful as a volunteer. Shortly after beginning her visits to the hospital, she became attached to a patient who had the same diagnosis and physical appearance as her husband. When the patient died the volunteer had a difficult time dealing with this second loss. It appeared that she had never given herself adequate time to get over her husband's death.

Volunteers may choose to work in a clerical capacity or to work directly with the patients: as a Unit Volunteer; Recreational Aide; Nutrition Cart Volunteer; Pastoral Care Assistant; Transporter, or a Friendly Visitor.

Volunteers perform tasks of "pleasure," too. We have volunteers who on Thursday nights bring cocktails to patients. This tradition was started in 1959. They may sing a song as well. On Monday evenings the Anchor Club (a group of retired Firemen) bring cocktails and entertainment to the patients.

There was once a request for a volunteer to sit with a patient who had no relatives and did not want to be alone. The volunteer got along well with this patient and as a result, after a while they became friends. As the patient's condition worsened, our volunteer arranged to stay with the patient for longer periods of time. When the patient died, our volunteer was there. This experience was in the hospital's best tradition; keeping promises and non-abandonment.

Calvary Hospital gratefully accepts the gift of time entrusted to the patients and staff by our Volunteers and makes every effort to honor this trust of their time and talents.

References

1. de Tocqueville A. Democracy in America. 2 volumes. New York: Vintage Books, 1958.

2. Dorang ES. AVNA organized hospice volunteer programs. Nursing Outlook:29(3)170-3.

PATIENT/FAMILY ADVOCACY
Joan Caldano

Calvary Hospital has always sought to welcome each patient as a person blessed with rights and privileges. In its mission and in its ministry, that same welcome is extended to the family and friends of the patient. As the patient enters the final phase of his/her life, there is a heightened urgency which calls not only for the utmost compassion but also for a degree of empowerment regarding health care and decision making.

Why would a sick person need to be empowered when we all know that hospitals are places where skilled professionals are about the business of healing? Yet it is that very phrase: the business of healing which has caused some patients untold difficulties as they move through a complex and oftentimes uncaring health care system.

The 60s and 70s saw technological advances, new medicines, new treatments and many more specialties developed. While these advances grew in size and complexity the very individuals who could most benefit from them were gradually being overwhelmed by this sometimes, impersonal technological giant called *"health care."* The family physician was overtaken by the specialist who more often than not concentrated his efforts in specific areas rather than the generalized well being of the patient.

So the dilemmas we confront include ... How does the individual make the institution work for him/her? How do we let the patient know that they, as consumers, have every right to expect the institution to work for them? How could these issues be addressed in order for the patient to enter into a collaborative effort with the physician and other health care professionals?

Long before these questions arose, Calvary Hospital had committed itself to maintaining a person-centered facility; a place where the health care of the patient is respected as well as his/her rights. Consistent with this commitment, the role of the Patient/Family Advocate was developed primarily to educate and support the patient's right to self-determination and freedom of choice. To that end the Patient/Family Advocate addresses the human needs and legal rights of each patient and/or family. In so doing, the Patient/Family Advocate sometimes acts as a spokesperson, exercising at the direction of the patient, powers which belong to the patient.

What "powers" or rights do patients have and how are they protected? In August, 1988, the New York State Department of Health took steps to address the issues of patient rights by mandating all hospitals to distribute a copy of the "plain English" Patients' Bill of Rights. Furthermore, it required the hospitals to provide inservice training to the patient care staff to assure their knowledge and understanding of patients' rights requirement; to post a copy of these rights in clearly viewed areas of the hospital; to designate a staff member to meet with each inpatient or their representative upon admission to explain these rights and provide information on how these rights can be exercised.

Calvary Hospital's response was immediate. In an effort to provide patient rights information so that the patient might understand and exercise these rights the Patient/Family Advocate Department was directed to meet and provide such information to each inpatient and/or the patient's representative upon admission. In addition, the Patient/Family Advocate was given the responsibility for coordinating efforts to address patient rights information for non-English speaking patients, as well as the vision and hearing impaired patient and/or family member.

Copies of Spanish, Italian, Chinese, Greek, Russian, French Creole, Yiddish, etc. Bills of Rights were sent to each hospital with suggestions as to how we might engage non-English speaking patients and families in conversations about care through interpreter services and devices for the vision and hearing impaired.

Telecommunication Devices for the Deaf (TDD's); Sign Interpreters; graphic Phrase Cards in Chinese, Korean, Russian, Spanish and Vietnamese; Braille Bill of Rights; ATT Language Line Services are examples of the devices in use at Calvary to enhance communication and disseminate information among staff, patients and family members.

A basic responsibility of the Patient/Family Advocate is to coordinate the effective response of the health care team with patients/family and broach issues which they may perceive as patients/families, impinging on their right to receive quality care. Ethical issues which arise around end-of-life decision making about the way to live and the way to die require a response from professionals which supports the involvement of patients and their families. In certain instances the Patient/Family Advocate calls together the Ethics Consult Team. This conglomerate provides a forum for the patient/family and members of the hospital Ethic's Committee whereby individuals are heard, issues are identified and ethical analysis of the issue is formulated. Other areas which require the intervention of the Patient/Family Advocate are the every day concerns of care, which, for the terminally ill, literally become "larger than life." When the patient/family empower the Advocate to act on their behalf, another type of mechanism is deployed.

The Advocate helps to identify the problem; addresses the parties involved; coordinates the interdisciplinary resolution with the same parties, reports back to the patient and ideally elicits satisfaction from the patient. These are two instances of Calvary's institutional interactions working for the patient within the system rather than abandoning them to the system.

Listening is a communication skill. While it is incumbent on the caregiver to provide information to the patient and/or family, it is as important to listen to what the patient and/or family has to say. The skill used here is the attentive, non-judgmental and non-interruptive style of focusing that allows the patient to speak his/her mind. Surprisingly, this style of listening sometimes permits an even greater understanding of peoples' backgrounds, their needs and their troubles. It gives meaning to the word compassion. In the absence of active listening, we create a climate where defensiveness, ignorance and anger can flourish.

Case Examples

I received a frantic phone call from a staff member at the hospital reception desk informing me that a family member of a patient about to be admitted wanted to go up to her room "right now," and "clean the walls!" I was perplexed and wondered if the staff person had heard correctly. Most emphatically, he insisted that he did. In fact, he had already come to the conclusion that something was a bit "odd" about this person making the request and reminded me that hospital policy and procedure would forbid this behavior.

Not one to let policy and procedure stand in the way of legitimate requests from patients or family members, I set out to meet this gentleman and hear for myself what was behind his request to wash walls. Trying to keep an open mind, I couldn't help but think that this could be just another one of those crazy requests that people expect the hospital to accommodate, e.g., organic lobster tails for the patient who wanted to eat nothing but! When I brought this gentleman into my office, I found him to be most gracious and quite articulate about his request, though somewhat annoyed over the encounter and treatment at the reception desk. After listening to him I found out that much was lost in the "translation" and judgments that both the individual and his need to wash walls were "crazy." Actually, this man's request was based on his mother's religious beliefs and his need to do everything possible to ease her transition to a facility for the terminally ill.

After sitting down, one on one, and focusing on what he was saying, I heard a son ask if he could go up to the room which would be assigned to his mother for the remainder of her days and pray! Pray, so that before his mother was placed onto her hospital bed, he would "cleanse" the room of the suffering spirit of the patient who had died in that room the day before. With the cooperation of the staff, the patient waited on her stretcher in the hallway outside the room while her son went inside to pray. As I closed the door to give him some privacy, I saw him get to his knees and with head bowed, clasp his hands silently in prayer. It struck me then, as I looked around at the ambulance attendants and the nurse, that we had gone from calling this man crazy to joining him in his prayer. We stood with our heads bowed, communicating in our own way. What could have led to confrontation had now been settled calmly and with increased awareness and sensitivity on the part of the care staff.

Another case in point:

Another similar incident taught us an important lesson about how to listen and understand a rather "brash, know it all" family member. By the time the hospital's admitting process was completed, this individual had managed to alienate most of the staff; attending and nursing staff were irate and insulted by her attitude toward them.

On the day of admission the niece of the patient came down to my office and in a lengthy monologue clearly stated that the entire admitting process including the medical and nursing assessment of the patient was objectionable. She belittled the attending by calling him a "know it all God" and had something to say about his attitude, approach, manner, care plan and medications. She also had a grievance about the admitting nurse. She proclaimed herself as a person who knows "exactly what is going on!" In fact, she took pride in the fact that she was quite adept at challenging the medical system and winning!

She backed this up with the story of her second heart surgery (at the same time her husband had just died.) She had studied the material used in the valve replacement and when the surgeon said he did not use this particular type she "fought" with him until he relented. She had won her battle! Clearly, the battle lines had been predetermined between a defiant family member and a vulnerable staff; all this within hours of admission! While I knew the patient would receive the best of care, I also realized this would pose a great challenge to staff because of the tense atmosphere established on the day of admission. When on the second day, this woman was back in my office complaining of inadequate treatment and care for her aunt, I knew some immediate intervention was necessary before this situation escalated. I invited her to sit down and talk to me about herself and she did, for quite some time without interruption. In essence, she told me that she was a "fighter" and would do anything to beat the system. She prided herself on this spirit by saying if she did not fight on her own behalf when her heart gave out she might not be alive today. After listening at some length to the niece's diatribes: the belligerence and contentiousness of her statements struck me as arbitrary, I was able to demise that she was no longer fighting her own battle but one for her aunt. Clearly, her frustration was being directed at the very people who were trying to do what ultimately she wanted for her aunt, that is relief from the symptoms of her cancer, of course to survive, and if not, some comfort in her final days. She paused, and with a deep sigh, sat back in the chair, looked me straight in the eye and said this was exactly what she was doing and promised from here on in "she would clean up her act!" The very next day the staff commented on a change in her attitude and for all intent and purpose the remainder of the hospitalization was uneventful.

In situations like this, it is easy to form judgments and label the individual as troublesome, so much so, that while care is maintained for the patient, encounters with the family member tend to become limited and stressful.

Autonomy and individualism, once buzz words for a "style" of compassionate care, are fully realized elements of Calvary's humanistic concern for the rights of the patient, family, friends, and staff.

PASTORAL CARE
Mary T. O'Neill

Care of the whole person is integral to Calvary's plan for each patient. Spiritual care -- care at the deepest level of a person's being -- is the specialty of the Department of Pastoral Services. It is care at the core of a person's relationship with self, with others and with God. Spiritual caregivers, i.e., chaplains, are concerned with the total person: the interdependence of mind, body, and spirit. Patients are met by a chaplain soon after their admission to Calvary, and the range of services (with respectful attentiveness to the needs of their spirit) are made known to them. This relationship is the foundation of the Calvary Mission and philosophy of nonabandonment and attention to the dignity of the person. Also, the patient is given the utmost respect and dignity to his/her very last breath. This goal is reflected by the love, care, and acceptance of the chaplain as the person moves towards greater peace and readiness for death. The chaplain has the privileged and sensitive task of assisting in the unfolding of this mystery at the most critical and most sacred moments of life.

The chaplains seek to convey the peace and love of God for each patient, believing that spiritual healing and growth are possible for all people regardless of their medical situation. When coping with the issues and concerns of illness and impending death, we offer ourselves and the resources of our faiths to be with people in their spiritual and emotional pain. This process is encouraged through spiritual conversation, prayer, sacraments, worship, counseling, and attentive presence. A person may or may not choose to confide in the chaplain, but a chaplain is always available to be an active listener or presence for that person.

To share another's faith is important and holy work. Therefore, members of the Department of Pastoral Services are trained professionals, endorsed by their faith groups for ministry in this interfaith environment of Calvary. Chaplains share in the hospital's educational mission, contributing both to the training of interns and staff members within the hospital.

Our interfaith Chapel offers Catholic, Jewish, and Protestant services. The patients can attend these services or watch them on their personal televisions. At other times, inspirational and relaxation tapes are televised through the in-house chapel channel, as an alternative to the commercial TV stations.

It is the policy of Pastoral Service to honor and secure at all times, the integrity and confidentiality of the chaplain's relationship with patients. Chaplains are encouraged to pray with their patients while being consistent with the religious beliefs of the particular person. Evening and morning prayer over the paging system are inclusive of the religious diversity of Calvary's population.

Each patient is visited regularly by members of the Department of Pastoral Services at times of distress, crisis, critical condition, and death. It is the responsibility of the chaplain to assess and treat the spiritual aspects of coping with illness, loss, dying, and death. These include the levels of spiritual pain identified as concern, distress, and despair. Obviously, the family members can feel intense spiritual pain and helplessness at this time also and their spiritual needs are no less important than those of patients. Spiritual concerns are identified when individuals present the desire and ability to cope with spiritual problems. There is no one whose life's meaning and goals are not somewhat challenged and called into question at the news of any serious illness, especially when this is life threatening. There are readjustments of relationships and belief systems, and a need to find meaning in the new circumstances that present themselves. "Whatever happened?" "I can't face this." "How can I get through this?" "What does it all mean?" Ministry at this time means helping them stay with the questions, articulate their feelings and assist them in searching for their answers within or in being peaceful with the questions themselves.

Spiritual distress results from the individual's difficulty in applying prior beliefs and values to this new circumstances. This can include a sense of meaninglessness and upheaval of values, hopes, dreams, and feelings. Questions regarding moral ethical issues, guilt, shame, regret can truly wear a person down and cause intense suffering. Patients and family members may feel varying degrees of anger and free-floating anxiety. They may be ashamed of the intensity of their anger at God, for example, and may not know how to deal with this or even talk about it. A sensitive chaplain will encourage them to express what's truly going on, authenticate their feelings, acknowledge the depth of that pain and hopefully help them emerge through their tears, grief, and fears to a place of hope and peace. One patient, for example, was the humorist of his social circle. He felt that, as a patient, he had to maintain that image with his family and visitors. However, he could express with the chaplain his outrage that God had allowed this to happen to him. His daughter was horrified at his expression of anger until the chaplain explained the appropriateness of his feelings. His daughter could then understand that he needed to express his "negative" and "humorous" feelings, and even, with help, she could encourage him to vent his rage. Because of this, an intimacy the father and daughter could not reach before was now accessible to them both. Being able to be part of this experience deepened their relationship. The patient died very peacefully and his daughter was left with the memory of an intimate connection with her father in his last days.

Spiritual despair, felt as utter darkness, meaninglessness, and hopelessness, is intense and deeply painful. A patient who has written books on death, for example, knew all there was to know, but when facing this pain, was rendered immobile and paralyzed with fear and hopelessness, and so her isolation increased. She didn't trust anything or anyone to help her and felt beyond help. Fidelity to visits and acceptance of her anger and orneriness were reminders of the willingness of others to be with her, and their availability to her when she was ready to let them into her uncharted terrain of feelings and spirituality.

In this period of preparation for death, people can learn some of life's most important lessons. People who have lived busy lives, filled with the challenges of family and work, too easily do not find time for the nurture of their spiritual self. However, a very ill person, especially one facing the end of life, can hardly avoid the questions of life's meaning and direction. They may have had a spiritual void in their lives that needs to be awakened and enlivened. It can be a significant source of support and strength for them. One young woman, for example, came to the hospital full of desperation at the thought of leaving her young children. She could not articulate her pain or express her anger. She was in a very dark place. With some very attentive presence to her in her pain, she did say that one of the hardest things was that she would not see her children grow up, nor even see her oldest daughter receive her First Communion. Arrangements were made for a ceremonial communion for her daughter to take place at the hospital. The mother blossomed back into life because at least one of her fears was squelched as well as a spiritual need met. She then could address other unresolved issues and have some quality visits with her children in her remaining days.

The caring support of a chaplain helps to promote spirituality which develops and changes over a lifetime. This presence is most beneficial because it helps patients look at death so he/she can embrace and live life until death.

The Department is committed to offering high quality pastoral care, 24 hours a day, 7 days a week. Chaplains are also attentive to the needs of staff persons and respond whenever possible. A ten minute Wellness Program is offered to staff several times weekly to reduce tension and provide an opportunity for relaxation and reflection through guided imagery, music, movement, etc. Also, the department sends cards to all staff in times of crises and special occasions in order to assure them of support. Along with chaplains, many staff members pray for patients and together observe the results of this power of prayer; patients come to peace and acceptance, testified to by their changed outlook and lowered level of demand on all those involved in their care.

Calvary speaks strongly to life -- life 'til the moment of death. The dying teach us about living and the preciousness of health and relationships and attention to our own inner resources. We are more than daily reminded of the truth of George Melton's quote: "Of one thing I am certain: the body is not the measure of healing; peace is the measure of healing."[1] What more could we want for our patients, their families, or for ourselves, as we face the end of life.

Reference

1. McWilliams, Roger J. Life 101: Everything we wish we had learned about life in school but didn't. California: Prelude Press, 1991.

BEREAVEMENT SUPPORT SERVICES
Catherine R. Seeley

"Show us your sun, but gradually. Lead us from star to star, step by step. Be gentle when you teach us to live again." The front of the condolence card sent to the family of every patient that died at Calvary bears this quote by Nelly Sachs. It captures the notion of process fundamental in adjusting to life-changing events and, at the same time, characterizes the tenor of Calvary Hospital's many Bereavement Services.

Step by step, patients and their families are accompanied by our extraordinary experts of care and comfort through the end of the terrible disease that has brought all of us together at Calvary where, briefly, our paths intersect. But these paths do not part with death. The continuum of care extends beyond it through the process of bereavement in a variety of ways.

Because patients admitted to Calvary are in the end stage of cancer, there are approximately fifty deaths per week here. A Christian Memorial Service is offered on the 2nd Saturday of each month for families and friends of patients who died during the previous four weeks. A Jewish Service of Remembrance is held every two months for Jewish patients who died during the previous eight weeks. As indicated above, the families of all patients receive invitations to these Services. Refreshments are served after the Services and discussion groups are conducted in English and in Spanish. While adults are in group, a children's group is also held.

Most noteworthy is the number in attendance at these services. Sadly, the facility in which a person dies often becomes a negative symbol to many families, dictating to some that they not be driven past that building, or taken to that place should anything ever happen. Amazingly, Calvary's staff--by their consistent standard of excellence--regularly manages to transform a potentially negative symbol into the very positive symbol of a community of concern and care: people return here in large number. (Memorial Services average 200 attendees per month.)

There is a kind of visual therapy in entering a room of 200 others who have been on a similar journey at the same exact time when, secretly up until this time, one may have wondered if he or she has been the only one upon whom such sorrow has been pressed. This is a gathering of "those who know" and it is a balm that touches isolation: "I am not alone in this."

Neither must the bereaved acquainted with this facility nor those within the community at large be alone in their grief, since all of our programs are open to the public. What follows is a brief overview of those various offerings.

Bereavement Support Groups

Calvary's Bereavement Support Groups run several times throughout the year and are facilitated by a chaplain and a social worker. These groups currently run for six consecutive weeks and there is no fee. Participants must reserve a place in the group in advance and agree to attend each session.

Organized assistance for the bereaved predominantly has had two categories: decathexis and resocialization. Bereavement Support Groups and bereavement counseling are models of the first, while clubs and/or organizations for widowed people-- with their focus on socials, trips, Sunday brunches, etc.--model the latter. Both are to be valued.

For many, though, going from a Bereavement Support Group into the next available alternative of such a club or organization feels too much like a quantum leap and grieving persons claim they are just not ready for this level of socializing yet. To many it makes sense: being intensely otherly focused during a loved one's illness and death often effects a diminished sense of self. Without this beloved other present as a daily part of one's life, questions unfailingly emerge: "Who am I now?" "What will I ever do?" "How do people go on?" "What will help me survive this?" This, of course, is the introspective bent that grief produces. By way of it, a necessary time of reclamation is thus introduced in the grieving process.

Usually and, most often informally, a severed relationship will require reclaiming one's individuality; one's true identity. For example, the mere shift in pronoun -- from "we," "us," "our" to "I," "me," "mine" -- invites subtle adjustments in consciousness: What do I think? What do I want? What are my needs? That easy cushion of plurality is no longer there and the person, now alone, must genuinely represent only him or herself and, perhaps, do so for the first time in life. The old formula of decathexis> reclamation>resocialization must occur. Its inclusion in Calvary's bereavement services takes the form of a step-up program called Discovery.

Discovery

Formal grief assistance programs such as support groups and/or counseling help us to express and understand our grief. Discovering a "next step" in the process, gives clues on how to replenish lost energies. Not a support group, this eight week workshop continues the mending process by engaging the participant in a three-tiered program: Know Yourself; Befriend Yourself; and Express Yourself. This workshop will lead participants to greater self-understanding, body awareness/stress reduction and relaxation techniques and guide them in the healthy expression of emotions through creative arts. This program is not for the recently bereaved and all participants must have previously attended a bereavement support group.

While Calvary offers grief assistance and support to adults, it is also vigorously engaged in "helping little hearts mend." Certainly, if there are small children in a family, they will be feeling the recent death of a family member or friend either directly as their own loss, or indirectly by sensing and seeing the sadness in those around them. Calvary Hospital has included children in its special formula of care and comfort by offering an after school program for grieving children.

Precious Moments

Precious Moments is for children aged 6-11 years. While children are in session, an adult group is conducted for parents or guardians accompanying the children. Children who are willing to participate in the adult group, must be accompanied by a parent or guardian. This after-school program runs for eight consecutive weeks in two locations, one here at the Hospital in the Bronx and the other in Queens at our Home Health Agency office. The program is conducted on Mondays and Tuesdays with the original intention that this early-in-the-week placement would help to set the tone at home and in school. This has been a well played hunch; evaluations at the end of the program consistently indicate that there were notable differences in the children's behavior at home and in school.

The needs of grieving children have been so poignantly represented by the participants in our program that we feel compelled to represent them to the community at large, that all of us will become more deliberate in the attempt to help little hearts mend. Thus, two videos on children and grief are being readied for production this year, thanks to a very generous grant from the Al Smith Foundation. One video will be for direct use with the grieving child; the other will be an instructional video for adults to help them better understand the needs of grieving children and how they might better meet those needs with compassion.

It is our intention to be advocates for the grieving child. What better, more extensive way to do this than through educational systems? Mentors Through Mourning is the medium by which this is being accomplished.

Mentors Through Mourning

Mentors Through Mourning is a Teacher Education Program in Childhood Bereavement offered by Calvary Hospital to administrators, teachers, guidance counselors, and social workers associated with elementary education. Sadly, it remains true that in the very environment equipping children to face the future--our schools--the most important lesson of all, coping with the death of someone they love, remains largely unaddressed and frequently ignored. This, because many adults do not recognize or understand the needs of grieving children or some of the most basic tenets of the grieving process. Mentoring educators with Calvary's expertise in bereavement will ensure that on site faculty personnel will be available to share with children the invaluable skills of adjustment and survival. Our goal is that every school in the New York metropolitan area will have at least one representative who will have been trained by Calvary to be a Mentor Through Mourning for the grieving children who will surely pass through their doors. This eight week program runs twice a year.

Because our Bereavement Support Groups are general bereavement groups, we offer evening lectures throughout the year that address specific losses under the New Horizons Program.

New Horizons Program

Special evening lectures, open to the public and free, are offered in an attempt to educate the community about grief-related issues. "Handling The Holidays," "Family Tree/Broken Branch: Death of A Sibling," "End of An Era: Adults and the Death of a Parent" are a few of the topics that address specific losses. A more formal educational program is the annual ten week Bereavement Course offered in the Fall.

The Calvary Hospital Annual Fall Bereavement Course

A ten-week course on bereavement and grief-related issues is offered to persons in the helping professions. This year eighty enrolled in the course with a typical composite profile of nurses, social workers, psychologists, clergy, group facilitators, chaplains, and parish ministers. Beginning in October, each evening session is two hours per week. Topics covered include Health and Grief; Patterns of Crisis Behavior; Grief Resolution and Contributing Factors; Personality Types; Children and Death; Spirituality and Grief; Multi-Cultural Aspects of Grief; Role of Interviewer/Models of Intervention; Special Issues; Homicide, Suicide, AIDS; Techniques, Rules and Dynamics of Running a Group. This course is not for the recently bereaved. Registration in advance is recommended. There is a fee for this course.

Calvary Hospital may be a small star in the constellation of health care, but its light is brighter than most. To the bereaved traversing through the "valley of darkness," its standard of excellence shines on all leading them gently through grief, "step by step."

HOME CARE
Carol Townsend and Anthony R. Riario

Home care is not only for the patient who no longer qualifies for inpatient care but also for those who wish to be at home even when risks are high. A proper home care program can assume most of the services rendered in the hospital or the nursing home when there is a highly motivated patient and family.

The Calvary Certified Home Health agency (Home Care Department) began in 1986 and was designed to offer patients and caregivers the full continuum of Calvary inpatient services at home. It has helped to reduce the hospital length of stay, improve the continuity of care, reduce the need for hospitalization, and produce better patient outcomes. One of its goals is to permit patients to remain home, if they wish to. The Program mirrors the in- and outpatient care by providing the same professional services. Patients can be readmitted to the hospital any time it becomes necessary.

All inquiries about Home Care Services are answered by experienced home care coordinators (registered nurses.) Direct contact with a health care professional assists referrers in planning and developing a safe, medically approved, comprehensive care plan. For hospitalized patients requiring extensive discharge plans, the home care coordinators meet with the discharge planner, patient and primary caregiver to arrange all the services needed to maintain the patient's safety at home. The home care physician is available at all times.

Community health nurses are essential members of the team. They provide direct primary care, total case management, and develop a one-to-one relationship with the patient. Clinical changes are noted and evaluated by the same professional. Twenty-four hour availability of community health nurses insures continuity of care.

Social workers provide assessments of the social and emotional factors related to the patient's illness. They evaluate the need for care, response to treatment and adjustment to care followed by care plan development. Community resource planning includes education, advocacy, referral, and linkage. This has become an important concern as individuals try to maintain desired lifestyles while combating the stress of illness and potential financial instability. Goal-oriented short-term therapeutic counseling is directed toward management of the illness, reactions and adjustment, strengthening the family system and trying to resolve conflicts related to the illness. Everyone appreciates this input into the treatment plan.

The patient's primary physician maintains a vital role on the interdisciplinary team and this role has increased. The physician expands the nurse's clinical knowledge and both contribute to the total management of the patient.

Patients in the community confined to their homes or without consistent medical supervision are offered home visits by the Calvary physician. They may also utilize our

Outpatient Department. The Calvary home physician has, at times, become a facilitator between the primary care physician and specialists involved in the patient's treatment plan. This continuity enhances the visibility of the program within the community.

Because many of our patients are fragile and experience decreasing mobility, other support services such as physical, occupational and speech therapies are also vital. These services focus on improving patients' ability to achieve maximum capabilities in daily living. It is particularly important that the physical therapist provide guidance and instructions for the patient and family in proper transfer techniques and safe utilization of assisting devices and equipment.

A registered dietician also makes home visits, attends inter-disciplinary team meetings, and advises the caregivers on the best means of providing nutrition.

Certified Home Health Aides, trained in assisting patients in activities of daily living and personal care provide a vital service to the patient. The aide becomes the member of the team depended upon to maintain a loving and safe environment.

The home care chaplain visits patients who may be grappling with life issues related to impending death. These concerns may include guilt, reconciliation, abandonment, judgment, afterlife, value of one's life, belief in the creator's role in causing or healing illness, and trust. Some form of resolution is crucial in the patient's or family's ability to cope with the illness. Pastoral care helps accomplish this goal. The chaplain (bilingual in English and Spanish) visits patients of every religious denomination and culture. Visits include active listening, sacramental prayer, and discussion of spiritual questions and education. Theological issues, methods of prayer, meditation, and relaxation techniques are all introduced and often prove helpful in reducing pain and anxiety. When necessary, the chaplain will contact a clergy person of the patient's faith for follow-up and will assist in obtaining religious articles, audio cassettes and in any other way possible. Other community resources such as support groups are contacted on request. The chaplain follows up all patients admitted to Calvary Hospital.

A memorable experience was that with EWR, a sixty-four year old woman who was diagnosed with carcinoma of the breast seven years prior to admission to Calvary. She had metastases to bones and meninges and was quadriparetic. The care in the hospital was intense and when she appeared to have achieved a relatively stable status, both she and her husband wanted to try to care for her at home. She remained home for five months before being readmitted to the hospital. Preparation for discharge was complex and required input from everyone -- the patient, her husband, her daughter, and every member of the interdisciplinary team.

The patient had concerns about returning home since the care in the hospital involved two aides to transfer her from a hospital bed to a special Lumex recliner. Her schedule for medication usage and problems with seizures further added to the anxiety of returning home. Nevertheless, she wanted to be there. The initial care plan established was that:

> The community health nurse would visit three times weekly to monitor disease progression and compliance with medications.
>
> The patient and her husband were carefully instructed about safety measures.
>
> The social worker would visit twice a month to assist with community resource planning and long term counseling for the husband and daughter.
>
> The home health aide would be placed for seven days to assist with personal care, transferring from bed to chair and skin care to prevent pressure ulcers.
>
> Physical therapy was asked to evaluate the patient for safety equipment and instruct the family in its use.

The family participated in the development of this plan and the discharge from the hospital was accomplished without incident.

All members of the interdisciplinary team visited at some time. A telephone conference was always available to prevent anxiety and the primary nurse was always available for these calls. The staff reassured the family that re-hospitalization could occur whenever necessary.

With progression of disease, her confusion increased, mobility decreased, and pain control required frequent evaluation and change of medications. Immediate readmission to Calvary was necessary during the night. An ambulance was obtained and the patient returned to the hospital accompanied by her husband. The patient survived for three weeks. Her death was due to hypercalcemia, thrombocytopenia and overall disease progression. Her family was at her bedside when she died. Those last months at home were a gift that could not have been given, without the extraordinary care and devotion of the home care team.

References

1. Neal A. The cultural basis of inadequate care. Health Progress 1996;77: pp 50-51.

2. Rich R. Home health nursing practice: concepts and application. 1992. St. Louis: C.V.M. Mosby.

3. Wendt D. Building trust during the initial home visit. Home Health Care Nurse 1996; 14: pp 92-98.

EUTHANASIA
James E. Cimino

The suffering experienced by those diagnosed as having a fatal illness can be overwhelming. We now have the skills to prolong life, but in so doing may also prolong the suffering. Society, in general, has become more sensitive to this problem as more value is being placed on the ethical principles of autonomy and justice. There is an increasing discussion of choices and dilemmas that arise at the end of life. When death occurs quickly the suffering befalls those who are left behind. They must deal with loss, grief and bereavement. These are burdens enough for the survivors. During the process of chronic illness, there is much more: the pain, the other physical symptoms, the denial, the anger, the bargaining, the depression, the hope, the disappointments, the abandonment of both the patient and the survivors. Other concerns are financial burdens and inability to understand the legal and ethical implications involved in achieving relief of suffering. I want to address one major controversy - the perception that euthanasia and suicide should be a sometime solution to this suffering.

Obviously, the most effective way of dealing with these problems would be to cure the underlying sickness. When the patient is in the terminal phase of illness, care should concentrate on the relief of symptoms. Yet, rarely do the parties involved entirely let go of the possibility of a new therapy or even a miracle that will cure the disease. This hope in itself is often linked with the terrible suffering. In spite of this, there is less often a call for early death but rather a hope that the miracle will occur. The goal of the hope requires redirection from longevity to fulfillment of what time remains. The best possible quality of life must be sought.

I have been involved with the care of dying patients during my entire medical career. In the early days of Hemodialysis, I struggled with the ethical quandary of how to select those patients who should be chosen to benefit from a new therapy that was only marginally available. In short, we were asked to decide who should live and who should die. During the past thirty-six years, my work has been more closely identified with that of the care of advanced cancer patients in the final stages of life. It is this background that helped frame my thoughts on euthanasia.

Non-Abandonment

The "abandonment syndrome" begins when the caregivers believe nothing can be done. It is emotionally and medically devastating to the patient and can lead to scientific blunders for the caregivers. There is *never* a time when nothing can be done. *Never.* In this book the chapters, *Intercurrent Diseases* and *Non-cancer Related Pain in End-of-Life Cancer Patients*, address the dangers to the patients when they are labeled as "terminal."

There have been too many similar events in all our hospitals. Physical abandonment leads to intellectual abandonment, inappropriate decisions and then, disaster. Therapeutic decisions in near end of life care must be made with the same careful deliberation that we apply earlier in the course of a patient's illness. I have cared for many patients who wished to give up prematurely until we addressed a symptom or concern that had been causing severe distress. Being ill is a frightening experience and having a fatal illness enhances this fear. Care in a hospital can be so impersonal that it adds to this trauma. *NON-ABANDONMENT* goes beyond the usual standards of legal negligence. It means removing this aura of fear. You must encourage communication, show genuine concern, be available, keep your promises, and ensure the patient's continuity of care. Throughout the terminal period, caregivers must be ever alert to aspects of clinical care which are reversible and if properly managed, will extend comfortable life. Symptom control is extremely important in these patients, but it cannot be used as an excuse for careless medical management. Competence and good clinical judgment are no less important here than in other areas of medicine. Caregivers should never "give up" trying to relieve symptoms. Patients can respond.

The designation of terminal can be misleading and requires explanation. A study of 301 physicians who responded to a questionnaire asking them to define "terminally ill" generally agreed that death would occur in six months or less. The Medicare Hospice program also uses a six-month life expectancy as a requirement for insurance coverage. I define it further, not only in time but also in clinical needs. To me, a terminal illness is a condition of progressive deterioration easily noticeable to experts. The patient requires assistance in activities of daily living. Death will eventually result because effective medical intervention is not available. Projecting the time of death is itself not a necessary criterion but in practice is usually thought of in terms of hours, days and weeks rather than months or years. The patient must *not* be classified as terminally ill except in the light of the best scientific knowledge.

Palliative Care

Palliative care is the active total care of patients whose disease is not responsive to curative treatment. Control of pain and other symptoms with attention to psychological, social and spiritual problems is paramount. The goal of palliative care is achievement of the best possible quality of life for patients and their families. It offers a support system to help patients live as actively as possible until death. The support system helps the family members cope during the patient's illness and in their own bereavement. Radiotherapy, chemotherapy and surgery have a place in palliative care provided that the symptomatic benefits of treatment outweigh the disadvantages.

Hospice

Hospice care provides aggressive comfort care in a patient oriented setting. For some period of time the patient may be hospitalized to solve problems that cannot be accomplished at home. Hospice itself is a philosophy of care rather than a place that incorporates palliative care. It addresses the psychological stability of both the patient and family during the illness and extends through the bereavement period. Calvary Hospital's program is founded on kindness, and the philosophy of non-abandonment and includes all the goals of Hospice.

Ethical Considerations

Ordinary or proportionate means of preserving life are those that in the judgment of the patient offer reasonable hope and benefit and do not entail an excessive burden or impose excessive expense on the family or the community. It is generally felt that a person has a moral obligation to use ordinary or proportionate means of preserving his or her life. The provision of nutrition and hydration is presumed to be a minimal or ordinary means of providing care and therefore, obligatory as long as it is of sufficient benefit to the patient and does not cause undue burden.

Extraordinary or disproportionate means are those that in the patient's judgment do not offer a reasonable hope and benefit or entail excessive burden or impose excessive expense on the family or the community. A person may forego extraordinary or disproportionate means of preserving life.

Ethical deliberation is the application of a moral code in a logical manner. While it is not necessarily legal, justice should be its foundation. Those involved in health care are different from their patients only in their obligation to be expert in their particular disciplines. Both the patient and the caregiver should behave ethically. Our goals should be to preserve life, relieve suffering and to do no harm while achieving these goals. When caring for the terminally ill, the standards for making ethical decisions should be no different from what they would be when caring for all patients - appropriate medical indications and the wishes of the patient. Care that is known to be futile is inappropriate. For most of us, these standards are rooted in the philosophies of Western civilization and the Judeo-Christian code of morality. Only in this context will we be able to agree on reasonable standards of care. Different cultures may require different explanations. These considerations are based on the principles of justice, beneficence, nonmaleficence, patient autonomy, the right of truth disclosure, priority (even sanctity) of life, quality of life issues, benefits to the patient proportionate to the burdens of intervention, the specific obligations of the health caregiver and hopefully, the avoidance of "slippery slope" decisions. Informed consent does not mean convincing the patient to do what we want, but rather for the patient to make an informed decision based on all the facts available.

Futility

The definition of futility is widely misunderstood and difficult to define. The same 301 physicians who were asked to define "terminally ill" were asked, "Regarding a terminally-ill patient, I consider a treatment 'futile' if the likelihood of success is ---- percent or below."[1] Most of the respondents thought 1-10% with a median and mode of 5% and a range of 0% to 60%. I try to avoid this term unless the likelihood of success is 0%. Rather, I discuss the entire concept of possible benefits to the patient.

Suffering

Although the fear of death and dying are usually considered as one, they are different. All of the following must be considered: the unknown, doubts, finality, regrets, guilt, sense of retribution, suffering during the dying process, anticipated grief, sorrow, loss of capacity, loss of control, depression, being a burden to others, loneliness, despair, inability to cope, denial, anger and bargaining, and finally, the instinct of self preservation.

Suffering encompasses all of these stated emotions and includes all the physical aspects of suffering such as pain, shortness of breath, loss of appetite, nausea, weakness, constipation, confusion, and dehydration. The physical signs of suffering can usually be addressed with a significant degree of success. It is the other emotions which are more difficult to relieve and require a great deal of time and commitment on the part of the caregiver. It is essential that time be spent in understanding the patient. Sometimes just being there is enough. It is essential that their suffering be acknowledged and they be reassured that they will not be abandoned.

Euthanasia and Suicide

The terms euthanasia and suicide are highly charged words and are often defined by a prejudged bias. Euthanasia generally means the deliberate, rapid, painless termination of life of a person afflicted with an incurable and progressive disease that is leading to death. It is considered by most in the category of suicide. It is different from withholding or discontinuing therapy and it is different from symptom control. In the Ethical and Religious Directives for Catholic Health Care Services[2], euthanasia is an action or omission that of itself or by intention causes death in order to alleviate suffering. It is this difference in defining euthanasia that often creates conflict in interpreting the act. Suicide refers to the willful act of causing one's own death.

A Right To Die

What if we are unable to completely relieve the symptoms to the patient's satisfaction? Is there a right to die? Are suicide and euthanasia a choice? This depends very much on the patient's own ethical, moral and religious values. For those who believe in the sanctity of life, where life is a gift and the person a steward of that life, euthanasia is almost always out of the question. For those who do not hold these values, the concept of rationale suicide is elusive and controversial. A pioneer in the study of suicidal behavior, Edwin Shneidman, captured this quality when he said, "It is not a thing to do while one is not in one's best mind. Never kill yourself when you are suicidal."[3] Even advocates for euthanasia agree that the decision should be made only when a person's judgment is intact and every effort has been made to treat underlying depressive illness. It is often a cry for attention and further help. Studies of suicide have found that 90 - 100% of the victims die while they have a diagnosable psychiatric illness. Suicide is rare in advanced cancer patients. Drs. Yeates Conwell and Eric D. Caine from the University of Rochester reported in the New England Journal of Medicine in October 1991, that of 85 suicides they had studied during the process of psychological autopsies (reviewing all of the information about the patient leading up to the suicide) only one victim had a diagnosed terminal illness.[4] Another study showed that of 44 patients in the latest stages of cancer only three had seriously considered suicide and each of them had a severe clinical depression.[5] Suicide, therefore, appears to be the result of an abnormal and likely treatable abnormality. When patients do not suffer a clinical depression (which should be treated if present) and sense they can still have control over their own care, they can usually tolerate most of the suffering.

Conclusion

Most symptoms can usually be ameliorated. Perfectly? - no, but enough to enable the patient to continue to live and die a natural death. When the fear of death itself is the most uncomfortable symptom experienced, suicide is certainly no answer for that. When it is the dying process itself, caregivers must work harder to help the patient. In order to minimize misunderstanding it is essential that the patient, the family and the caregivers redefine what the goal should be. Should it be relief of suffering or death?

Finally, a very important prohibition in the argument against euthanasia is the potential for abuse. Who is unable to tolerate the suffering - the patient, the caregivers, the family? We should understand that even if one considers euthanasia and suicide as ethically permissible, the potential for errors and abuses can be too great a price for society to pay.

Aside from the sanctity of life arguments, my objections to euthanasia are based on the pervasive instinct of self (life) preservation, the finality of death leaving no room for error, the evidence that suicide is likely due to a treatable abnormality and the potential for abuse. The ultimate solution may never be perfect. However having control, completing clear advanced directives, seeking comfort care and understanding that comfort care which may lead to unintended shortening of life, is generally considered ethical, moral and permissible, will make the suffering more tolerable. When we fail to relieve suffering and also deny a request for euthanasia, our obligations, as our *brothers' and sisters' keepers*, is what will define our humanity.

References

1. Van McCrary S, et al. Physicians' quantitative assessments of medical futility. J Clin Ethics. Summer 1994; pp 100-105.

2. Ethical and Religious Directives for Catholic Health Care Services November 1994; No. 60, p 23.

3. Shneidman ES. Some essentials of suicide and some implications for response. In: Roy A, ed. Suicide, Baltimore: Williams and Wilkins 1986: pp 1-16.

4. Conwell Y, Caine ED. Rational suicide and the right to die. N Engl J Med 1991; 325: pp 1100-1103.

5. Brown JH, et al. Is it normal for terminally ill patients to desire death? Am J Psychiatry 1986; 143: pp 208-211.

ASSISTED SUICIDE
Michael J. Brescia

Nationally health care has taken on both a political and an economic urgency to adopt cost-saving measures, especially at the end of life where medical expenditures may escalate rapidly. Independent health insurance plans and managed care payers have great reluctance to allocate funds for advanced cancer when therapy is considered symptomatic and palliative. However, the control of suffering is not an economical event. It requires staff, professional and paraprofessional, along with the complex administration of drugs and preventive measures to preclude a painful and protracted clinical course.

Frustration and failure in reducing health care costs, along with society's abandonment of the suffering, incurable patient, have prompted active discussion of physician-assisted suicide, and even explicit assent in certain public arenas. Of greater concern may be the implicit assent in some legislative bodies.

The ultimate cost-saving measure is physician based and controlled assisted suicide. Across the land, in our homes and our nursing homes, in mini vans, cellars, trailers and even reverently in our churches, physician-assisted suicide, with governmental consent, can become a legal cost-saving health care policy, which suits the expedient and morally bereft mind set.

I read with despair the finding that placing a nozzle over the exhaust system of an automobile, and pumping carbon monoxide into a patient's lungs, is a form of compassionate medical therapy for incurable disease, as long as it is requested by the suffering recipient.

At Calvary Hospital, there is a scientific and humane alternative to the organized, cooperative, final exit of incurably ill cancer victims. Calvary Hospital, by its mission, sees in every suffering patient a supreme dignity, even in the confines of a decaying body.

Approximately 2,500 cancer patients are admitted to Calvary Hospital each year. Almost all are suffering from wasting due to incurable cancer. The average length of stay is 25 days. Over 90% of these patients die.

Patients are admitted with cancers that have robbed them of their aspirations and futures. These tumors have stolen their lungs, disfigured their faces, silenced their voices, broken their bones, and paralyzed their extremities. Many have been rendered hairless, wasted, helpless, dependent, and bedridden. Often they vomit, bleed, swell, and become deformed. They never are abandoned. Never do they feel the absence of love, and never have our patients asked for physician-assisted suicide. Considering their terminal clinical afflictions, Calvary Hospital should be besieged with requests for assisted suicide and become a killing field for doctors of medicine. Yet, neither are we requested to assist in suicide, nor do our patients despair.

The major problem with our current social structure is the apparent inability to understand the nature of suffering. Hence, the solutions are expedient; or over simplified; driven finally to argue for the rapid dispatch of the afflicted reminders of our own mortality; falsely clothed in the moral platitudes of mercy, choice and dignity. There is no dignity with a plastic bag tied over one's head and drowning in one's own spittle and emesis within the confines of a rusted mini van.

Suffering is an interrelated system of thoughts and emotions, which is far more complicated than physical pain alone. Suffering involves a complex mix of the spiritual, mental, emotional and physical components which completes a human being. At Calvary Hospital, the unremitting goal is the commitment to relieve suffering in all its faces.

When the discussion of medical care in terminal illness involves physical symptoms alone, the entire notion of suffering is confounded. Suffering involves much more than physical pain. The physical aspects of pain are rapidly and effectively controlled by a skilled staff of physicians and nurses. We have no problem controlling physical pain.

Spiritual pain begs for the connection of man to God and God to man. Mental pain involves anxiety, agitation, sadness, depression, and even confusion and delirium.

Emotional pain is indeed the most resistant form of suffering and can be treated only by other humans who are committed to be the physical presence at the bedside.

Emotional pain begs for the presence of other feeling people. Emotional pain involves the final farewell to spouses, families and friends; the recognition that a life may be unfulfilled; the knowledge that children will not be seen to adulthood; that grandchildren will never be known. The earth is a great glass globe in which other humans have futures which may never be shared. Patients feel powerless, betrayed by the body, abandoned by man and forsaken by God; peering into a world they may no longer enter. During these periods of reflection, the emotional pain may become insufferable and unbearable.

It is during these periods that victims may ask for assisted suicide. Only immersion of our patients in a sea of love can control the emotional pain. We simply hold, caress, nurture and surrender to our patients all that we humans can give to another. Indeed, we wait with them in the vestibule of another world and let go when a love greater than our own pulls them free.

We do not have requests for physician-assisted suicide, in an arena where such requests should abound. Calvary Hospital has treated many thousands of cancer patients. We are a scientific and social experiment which answers one of the most pressing issues of our time.

We exist, here in New York, as a living, magnificent monument to physicians and nurses and all caregivers treating patients who need them the most when they would suffer the greatest.

Indeed, we are a treasure in this health care system. Now we may be the beacon for a collapsing moral system.

PERCEPTIONS, DEPERSONALIZATION, REFLECTIONS - LITERARY CORRELATES IN PALLIATIVE MEDICINE
Anthony R. Riario

As physicians, we are accustomed to seeing ourselves as immune to illness, aging, imperfections. Recently, after visiting an acquaintance in a nursing facility, my self-perception was shaken. Arno, whom I'd not seen for some ten years asked me, "Who are you? You've grown so old, I wouldn't have recognized you." This encounter led me to reflect on the stories of life, the literature I cherish that has helped me understand myself better, and the patients and the families I care for.

Stories are an integral part of existence. They elucidate, educate and entertain. Geoffrey Chaucer recounted the twelfth century pilgrim tales as they traveled to Canterbury, site of burial of Thomas Beckett, murdered in 1170. These tales helped people forget their misery, the plague deaths, the black death that had spread to England from Europe in 1347 killing some 25 million people. In his *Decameron*, Giovanni Boccaccio (Chaucer's Italian counterpart) used stories to help people laugh and forget their misery.

Camus used the plague as it affected a city in North Africa as a metaphor to help understand suffering. Rieux, the physician, tells us he became a doctor because he had to, because of an inner voice. And then he had to see people die. "Have you ever heard someone say 'never' to death. I have. And I just can't get used to that. But since death seems to rule our existence, wouldn't it be better if we didn't believe in God but rather fight death since God is silent in his heaven?"

"Yes, therefore, your successes are always transient," replies Tarrou, his friend.

"Yes, I'm aware of that but it's not reason enough to stop trying. Yet this plague is for me a never-ending failure."[1]

When we experience burnout, do we echo Tarrou's sentiment? Do we rather intellectualize our work, seeing suffering as a cleansing force, or are we like the country priest who ministers to the dying rather than trying to make sense of all their suffering?

A knowledge of literature may help to build a bridge with patients when we share a favorite story, or even a common time frame. Don't we often use neighborhood experiences as a basis for conversation? A physician may find a common bond with the patient when discussing a musical or literary experience.

Diego Velasquez, the 17th Century painter of the Spanish Court, painted some of the favorite dwarfs of the monarch, Philip IV. They stare at us from their portraits as human beings much like ourselves -- not as objects of derision or laughter. We must never forget that a human personality exists behind the ailing or natural exterior;

it may be waiting only for our love and comprehension to let it breathe. We need to communicate with these people, rather than shun them because they are different.

Per Lagerkvist in his novella, *The Dwarf* states, "I mentioned that my face was exactly like that of other men... it is very lined, covered with wrinkles, I do not look upon this as a blemish. I am made that way and I cannot help it if others are not. It shows me as I really am, unbeautified and undistorted . . . I think that the other faces are absolutely expressionless."[2]

As a metaphor for those misshapen by illness or birth or accident, this is a fierce cry for understanding. Consider the sick person with head and neck changes secondary to ablative surgery or illness. Do we view the patient as less than human?

Bill Becker wrote in 1985, "Why me? I'm a nice guy...Never threw sticks at someone's insecurities...never generated an intentional sadness. I used my talents. I lived my passions. Dealt with my weaknesses . . . It made me a growing, caring, thinking, vulnerable, mistake-making human (a nice guy). So, why me?"[3] -- before dying of AIDS.

Another aspect of illness, described in Jean-Dominique Bauby's *The Diving Bell and The Butterfly*, is depersonalization.

I can find it amusing, in my forty-fifth year, to be cleaned up and turned over, to have my bottom swiped and swaddled like a newborn's. The next day, the same procedure seems to me unbearably sad and a tear rolls down through the lather a nurse's aide spreads over my cheeks.

Already, they are wheeling me back, shivering, to my room, on a gurney as comfortable as a bed of nails. Having turned down the hideous jogging suit provided by the hospital . . . my old clothes could easily bring back poignant, painful memories . . . If I must drool, I may as well drool on cashmere.[4]

Is there not a better way to transport a patient than on those hospital "johnnies" that expose our nakedness, that relegate us to a dreary similarity to the other sufferers?

Tolstoy, in *Anna Karenina* describes Nikolai Levin's dying as follows:

Hitherto, each individual desire aroused by suffering or privation, such as hunger, fatigue, thirst, had brought enjoyment when gratified. But now privation and suffering were not followed by relief. 'Turn me over to the other side,' he would say, and immediately ask to be put back again. 'Give me some beef tea; take away the beef tea.'

While the priest was reading the prayers, the dying man showed no signs of life. His eyes were closed.

'He is gone,' said the priest, and made to move away; but suddenly there was a faint stir in the clammy moustache of the dying man, and from the depths of his chest came the words, sharp and distinct in the stillness:

'Not quite . . . soon.'[5]

Do we talk about the dying in a flippant, intemperate or inappropriate way, forgetting that hearing is one of the last senses to leave?

William Styron describes, in *Darkness Visible,* the ravages of depression on the psyche.

> The genetic roots of depression seem now to be beyond controversy. But I'm persuaded that an even more significant factor was the death of my mother when I was thirteen -- the death or disappearance of a parent, especially a mother, before or during puberty -- appears repeatedly in the literature of depression as a trauma sometimes likely to create nearly irreparable emotional havoc. The danger is especially apparent if the young person is affected by what has been termed 'incomplete mourning' - has, in effect, been unable to achieve the catharsis of grief, and so carries within himself, through later years, an insufferable burden of which rage and guilt and not only dammed-up sorrow, are a fact and become the potential seeds of self-destruction."[6]

Describing what he'd like from his doctor, Anatole Broyard wrote in *Intoxicated by My Illness*:

> I see no reason or need for my doctor to love me -- nor would I expect him to suffer with me. I wouldn't demand a lot of my doctor's time; I just wish he would brood on my situation for perhaps five minutes, that he would give me his whole mind just once, be bonded with me for a brief space, survey my soul as well as my flesh, to get at my illness, for each man is ill in his own way.

> Too often we act like automatons stripping the patient of his humanity -- he is a congested chest or a failing heart or renal insufficiency or a room number. The person cries out for healing, comprehension, and yes, at times, a smile. What about an exchange of reflections on literature, the joy of music, a baseball score ... the possibilities are myriad.

> My physician must be one not enamored of self, devoid of that sin of self-importance, of how great thou art; rather it is empathy that is at the cornerstone of the physician-patient covenant.[7]

Another capital sin is the arrogance of health, of omniscience of the caregiver -- the folded arms, the physical distance we observe from the patient. There is so much need to hold a hand, to spend some time with the patient, not just to cover the clinical aspects, but to enter into human relationships, to experience the hug, the hand-holding. A pastoral care person becomes specially valued here.

Some personal observations are echoed in *Screaming in Silence* from a midwest nursing home:

> Why do they talk about me as if I'm not here? I wish people would realize I'm mute, not deaf. I would tell the day shift aides to leave my TV alone and watch soap operas elsewhere. If I could talk, I'd tell them I don't like being called 'Gramps,' 'Pops' . . . 'Old Boy' any more than I like being referred to as 'the stroke in room 24.'

Certainly, A. Souffrant (a name I believe more descriptive than real), is a perceptive sufferer.[8] As for me, I would ask for the overhead lights to be turned off when I'm sleeping, not to use face masks for oxygen unless I'm comatose.

The quintessential question in palliative care is how do we die, how is the dying process? This is elegantly and amusingly described by Somerset Maugham in his last play, *Sheppey*. Sheppey, the barber of Jermyn Street, London has an encounter with death.

Sheppy:	Who are you?
Woman:	Death
Sheppy:	Well, I'm glad you've told me. I shouldn't have known otherwise. Sit down, won't you?
Death:	No I won't do that.
Sheppey:	In a hurry?
Death:	I have no time to waste. I'm not often welcome. And yet sometimes you'd think they'd be glad to see me.
Sheppey:	Look 'ere, you ain't come 'ere on my account.
Death:	Yes.
Sheppey:	You're joking. I thought you'd just come to 'ave a little chat. You must call again some other time.
Death:	I'm too busy for that.
Sheppey:	I don't fancy the idea of leaving this world. I know my way about and I'm at 'ome 'ere. Seems silly at my age to go on a wild goose chase like this.
Death:	Are you afraid? Are you ready then?
Sheppey:	To tell the truth . . . I don't feel like making a journey tonight.
Death:	It's an easy one.
Sheppey:	I won over 8000£ in the Irish sweep. It would be ridiculous for me to pop off just when I'm going to do a bit of good in the world.
Death:	It does happen like that sometimes. The world will get on quite well without you.

Sheppey:		You know, I don't feel at all well. I think I ought to see the doctor.
Death:		You'll feel better presently.
Sheppey:		There's one thing I'd like to ask you before we go. What's on the other side, really?
Death:		I've often wondered.
Sheppey:		Do you mean to say you don't know, taking people away, one after the other, young and old, whether they like it or not, and you don't know where it is they're going?
Death:		It's no business of mine.
Sheppey:		Which way do we go?
Death:		Out of the door.
Sheppey:		That seems rather tame, I thought we'd fly out the window or pop up the chimney. Something spectacular, you know... Well, I'll just put on my boots.
Death:		You'll have to come without.
Sheppey:		I shall look funny walking about without my boots on.
Death:		Nobody will notice.

Doesn't this dialogue from the play sound familiar to us in palliative medicine? We hear bargaining, cajoling, weariness, and the relief of death. Today's dying patient has been analyzed, scrutinized and dissected philosophically, clinically, and socially. The humanity of it all has too often been obscured.

REFERENCES

1. Camus A. The Plague. New York: Vintage International, 1957.

2. Lagerkvist P. The Dwarf. New York: Hill and Wang, 1945.

3. Becker B. An Immediate Desire to Survive. Bryn Mawr: Torrance & Co., 1985.

4. Bauby JD. The Diving Bell and the Butterfly. New York: Alfred A. Knopf, 1997.

5. Tolstoy L. Anna Karenina. New York: David McKay, 1992.

6. Styron W. Darkness Visible, A Memoir of Madness. New York: Random House, 1992.

7. Broyard A. Intoxicated By My Illness. New York: Clarkson Potter, 1996.

8. Souffrant A. Screaming in Silence. J Gerontol Nursing 1993:44.

9. Maugham, SW. Sheppey. London: William Heinemann, 1993.

EXPENDITURES FOR DYING PATIENTS: TOO MUCH OR NOT ENOUGH?
Frank A. Calamari

The intense debate currently underway in the United States concerning the reform of our health care delivery system has many complicated public policy and ethical dilemmas connected to it. None are more difficult to resolve than those surrounding the care and treatment of adults in the terminal phase of illness. Compounding society's difficulty in dealing with this issue are two major concomitant parameters - increasing technologic capabilities and decreasing moral and social standards. Without dwelling on the apparent moral and social degradation of the United States in recent years; it appears that every step forward that has been made (e.g., Civil Rights and Social Justice legislation), there have been two steps backward on many fronts (e.g., substance abuse, violent crime, illegitimacy rates, etc.).

Concerning the forces of technology, one has only to revisit the social and epidemiological conditions present at the turn of this century. Life expectancy in the United States for the average male was 48.1 years and the average female 51.1 years. Today those numbers have increased to 72.6 years and 79.3 years respectively.[1]

In addition, it was not uncommon for a hospital to discourage admission to many in need, including those people with terminal illness. Also, the academic training for physicians was in disarray and this led to doctors being ill equipped and poorly trained to treat serious disease.[2,3] How ironic it is, therefore, that at this time, with some of the finest academic and research centers in the world, whose physicians can perform "medical miracles" and extend life beyond the dreams of our forbearers, that we are confronted with some who either can see few bounds for technical intervention (*FUTILE CARE*) or those who would seek to deny prematurely even the most fundamental of interventions (*ABANDONMENT*). A most recent permutation of the latter includes the trend to popularize and legalize the ability of physicians to participate actively in assisted suicide employing starkly different approaches, criteria and philosophies.[4,5]

For many years now, pundits in the United States have "railed against" the amount of resources spent on dying patients, particularly during their last six months of life. Regretting the high cost of dying, some have estimated that between 27-30% of all Medicare funds (funds spent on people 65 years+) are spent on approximately 6% of Medicare beneficiaries who die in that year.[6,7]

Extrapolating Medicare data to the population in general has led many to estimate huge potential savings in this area. They contend that through the use of Advance Directives, Hospice care, and the education of futile therapies, tens of billions can be saved and redistributed to other pressing health care needs.[8] Interestingly though, when one examines and analyzes the most current data and then corrects some faculty baseline assumptions, a different picture emerges. For example, although the 6% of the Medicare population who do die do consume approximately 30% of

Medicare resources in that year, only 1% of the overall American population dies in that same year. Projecting straight line data from the Medicare population to the general population is misleading. Secondly, embedded in the data is the presumption that *all* the deaths identified were predictable. In fact, physicians report this is not doable, "Retrospective cost studies will inflate costs at the end of life as compared with costs for patients known in advance to be dying because they include many patients receiving expensive care who are not expected to die, yet do die."[9] In addition, reviewing the data on cost reductions associated with: the use of Advance Directives; delivering end stage care through a Hospice; and reducing "futile care," are far from conclusive or impressive. Data on patient bills, comparing those with Advance Directives vs. those without, show no significant difference.[10]

In terms of Hospice care compared to an acute hospitalization, costs are lower, but depending on whether the Hospice is home based or hospital based, the savings range from 27% - 15%;[11] significant but not huge. Finally, in the area of futile care an even more confusing and mixed picture emerges. To begin with, defining and identifying a futile action, even among physicians, is far from an exact science. In a recent study designed to measure the general level of agreement among physicians on the issue of futility, little agreement was actually found. Physician definitions of futility were divided into two groups: those focused on quality of life criteria, and those focused on psychological issues, including the psychology of the physician and the patient.[12]

Furthermore, when one considers the other side of the futility coin, namely, individual patient's needs, we also see little agreement. Depending upon the individual patient's clinical picture and psychological gestalt, what may be considered futile intervention for one patient could actually be indicated and appropriate for another patient. It appears that more research is required in this area and that the data on this subject is currently nonconclusive and perhaps even somewhat counter-intuitive.[13] The purpose of this elaboration is twofold: First to propose that, contrary to the declarations of some, the expenditure of resources for the dying patient may not be inappropriate, and secondly, money is not the main cause, nor is it the main solution, for the Abandonment/Futility issue. In general, it appears that patients are not abandoned because of lack of money, and futile care, although never desirable, does not seem to be bankrupting the system.

References

1. Schick R. Statistical handbook on aging Americans. Phoenix: Oryx Press, 1994

2. Flexner A. Flexner report on medical education in the U.S. and Canada. Washington Science and Health Publications, 1910.

3. Rosner D. Heterogeneity and uniformity historical perspectives on the voluntary hospital. In sickness and in health. A United Hospital Fund Book. New York: McGraw-Hill, 1994.

4. Quill TE, et al. Regulating physician assisted death. New Engl J Med 1994; Vol 331 (2): pp 119-123.

5. Kevorkian J. Prescription medicine: The goodness of planned death. Amherst: Prometheus Books, 1991.

6. Lubitz JD, Reilly GF. Trends in Medicare payment in the last year of life. New Engl J Med 1993; Vol 22, pp 1092-96.

7. McCall N. Utilization and costs of Medicare services by beneficiaries in their last year of life. Arch Intern Med 1992; Vol 152, pp 329-42.

8. Singer PA, Lowy FH. Rationing patient references and cost of care at the end of life. Arch Intern Med 1992; Vol 152, pp 478-80.

9. Emanuel EJ, Emanuel LL. The economics of dying; the illusion of cost savings at the end of life. New Engl J Med 1994; 330: pp 540-44.

10. Teno J, Lynn J, Phillips R, et al. Do advance directives save resources? Clin Res 1993;41:551A, Abstract.

11. Kidder D. The effects of hospice coverage on Medicare expenditures. Health Services Resources 1992; 27: pp 195-217.

12. McCray SV, et al. Physicians' quantitative assessments of medical futility. Jr Clin Ethics, 1994; pp 100-104.

13. Jakkimainen L, et al. Counting the costs of chemotherapy in a National Cancer Institute of Canada randomized trial in non-small cell lung cancer. J Clin Oncol 1990; Vol 8: pp 1301-09.

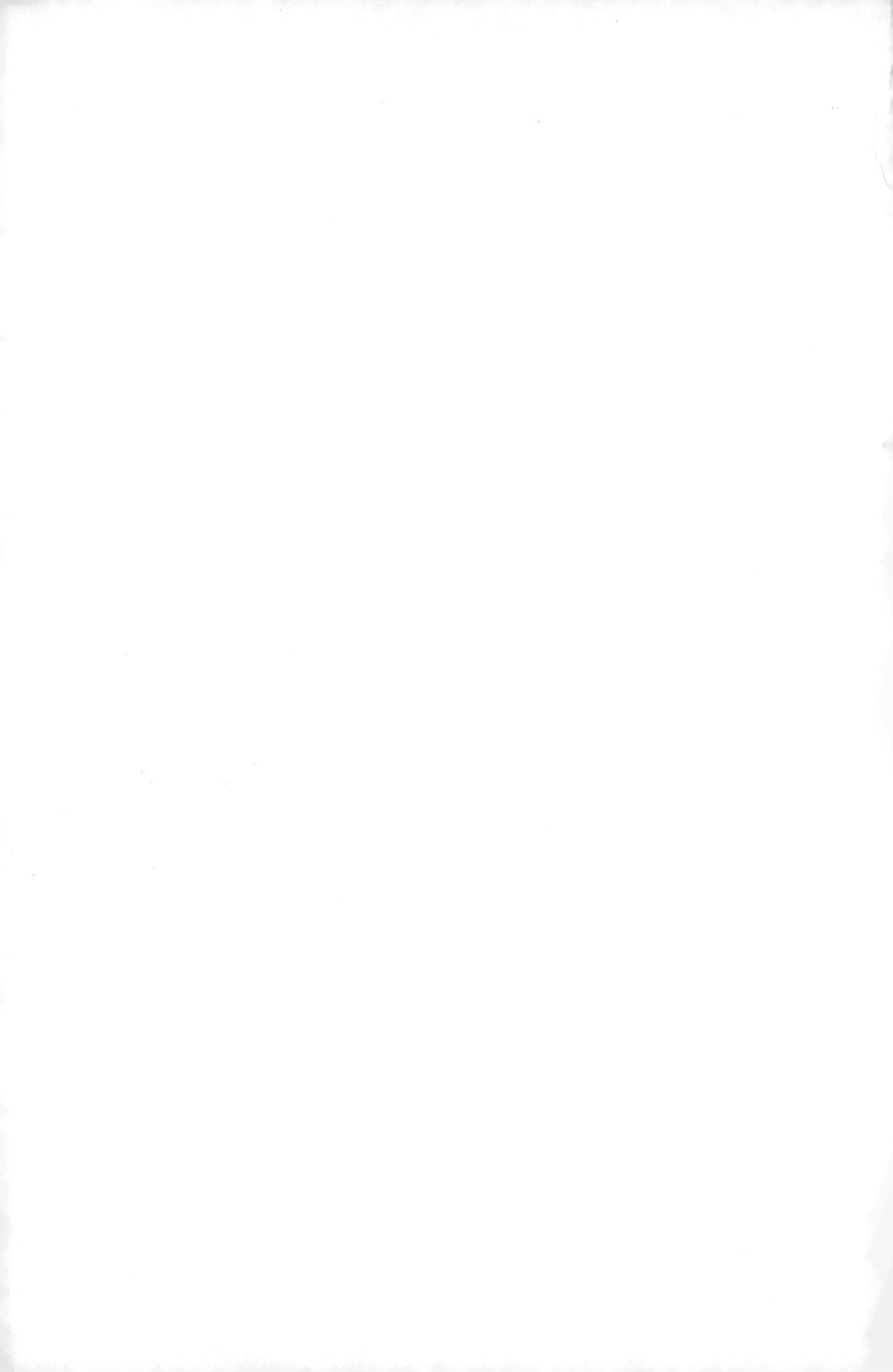